CHILD
OFFENDERS

PATTERSON SMITH REPRINT SERIES IN
CRIMINOLOGY, LAW ENFORCEMENT, AND SOCIAL PROBLEMS

A listing of publications in the SERIES *will be found at rear of volume*

PUBLICATION NO. 75: PATTERSON SMITH REPRINT SERIES IN
CRIMINOLOGY, LAW ENFORCEMENT, AND SOCIAL PROBLEMS

CHILD OFFENDERS

A Study in Diagnosis and Treatment

HARRIET L. GOLDBERG, LL.B., Ph.D.

Domestic Relations Court, Juvenile Court, Toledo, Ohio. Formerly Assistant Corporation Counsel assigned to the Children's Court of New York City

Montclair, New Jersey
PATTERSON SMITH
1969

Copyright 1948 by Grune & Stratton, Inc.
Reprinted 1969, with permission, by
Patterson Smith Publishing Corporation
Montclair, New Jersey

SBN 87585-075-8

Library of Congress Catalog Card Number: 69-14928

TO

Dr. Hertha Kraus of Bryn Mawr College,
an inspiring teacher and friend.

FOREWORD

THERE ARE few subjects that are at once more controversial and fascinating than what to do with a misbehaving child, the so-called problem child. Opinions and beliefs, expert and enthusiastically amateur, concerning the rearing of children, are as sharply divided and diverse as they are in politics and economics. Conservatives, liberals and radicals in this area of thought quarrel endlessly and, it sometimes seems, fruitlessly. As if there were not enough in this precarious world to bewilder the disturbed child and harassed parent, this conflict among representatives of the various behavior disciplines must further serve to confuse the guardians of the child's welfare in the home, the school, and community.

However, disagreement, even violent, is a sign that the science may be a dynamic one. Emerging from the debates, in a more tolerant and enlightened era behavior scientists will doubtless have reached a modicum of agreement on the differential diagnosis of disturbances; therapeutic techniques will have been developed which produce more conspicuous results than they do today. Psychometric devices or personality tests, psychiatric evaluation, and prediction tables, though they may lack the precise accuracy of an x-ray, will yet possess the ingredients of tools that are singularly free from the prejudices of one or another school of entrenched psychological or sociological thought.

Too, the behavior scientists of the future will know with greater clarity (because they will probe more deeply into it) that secret of human behavior we call *motivation*. More than ever before, we now know there can be no enduring benefit from treatment until we know more about cause. But opportunities to enhance our knowledge of causes are being wasted constantly and prodigally. It is a melancholy fact that in perhaps no other area of human activity in which children make contact with adults does the nonexistence of adequate tools for diagnosis and therapy become more evident than in the school. Yet it is there that the peculiarly personal traits and characteristics of children can be observed strategically. Aggressiveness, lying, exhibitionism, cheating, shyness, truancy and sexual irregularities are but a few on the lengthy roster of danger signs manifested in school. If the school had available devices for exploring the roots of characteristics which later blossom into hopelessly fixed patterns of antisocial behavior, such children could be treated in timely fashion. Under such conditions crime prevention could truly rise to the dignity of disease prevention.

Dr. Goldberg's rich experience with habitually truanting children possesses the significance of emphasizing how truancy is but one symptom of a deeper anxiety or disturbance that is all too rarely investigated—how superficially that symptom may be and often is regarded by school authorities as simply a police problem.

In the presently mysterious (to the public) process by which adjustment is shaped from maladjustment and emotional maturity is made to supplant a species of infantilism, the prevalent idea that rigid discipline, organized recreation, and sterile moral indoctrination represent effective treatment for the disturbed youngster, is daily being proved demonstrably fallacious. But if such devices are to be abandoned, it must be for better reason than that they are merely obsolescent. Mankind must probe and understand this secret of motivation before embarking on the delicate mission of therapy, especially for incipient behavior deviations.

A few words about how the pages which follow serve to bring us closer to an awareness of the early beginnings of antisocial behavior. Against the background of our past error, present uncertainty, and our groping for the whole scientific truth (if, indeed, that is ever attainable), this book is welcome. The author has had the wisdom to resort generously to the case-system, that pragmatic application of theories and principles to living people and actual episodes. To illuminate her text she has given us samples of day-by-day problems arising in a busy court. The principles of accepted, modern casework thus become transcendently clear when they are made to apply to the living, frequently ugly, situations in which children find themselves.

Hence, this collection of cases is a unique contribution to a growing literature. Convened within the covers of no other book, according to my recollection, will there be found cases so studiously sharpened to the revealing symptom of truancy, that tell-tale manifestation frequently appearing in the total constellation of antisocial behavior.

Moreover, Dr. Goldberg hammers out on the anvil of the readers' minds what all of us have been striving to impart to the public, namely, that we will not make substantial progress in the prevention of delinquency or the other manifestations of maladjustment until we ameliorate the conditions which inevitably produce those symptoms.

Without detracting from the soundness of what is here contained, there should be recognition of protests against the concept that truancy may be handled as a separate phenomenon, plucked from the mosaic of nonconforming behavior by, among other things, creating a separate court and staff to deal with it. In my opinion these protests are valid. Only by regarding the total personality of the child against the totality of his experiences will we ever move along toward more solid achievement in a field so far characterized by such dismal failure.

The book, therefore, should be a desk companion, a handy reference, a manual, for the neophyte as well as for the established practitioner in the difficult but fruitful field in which man struggles to understand and solve the problems of children. With it, the task may become easier; without it, it is my feeling that the literature would have been poorer.

A word of caution: what is here contained is not a self-operating mechanism. In the last analysis the value of this book—like that of every other work in this field—depends upon the use to which the reader puts the material herein embodied. Here it has been stored; it is for you to extract what is useful —and *use* it!

EDWIN J. LUKAS
Executive Director
Society for the Prevention of Crime

New York City
October, 1947

ACKNOWLEDGMENT

MANY people have contributed to the writing of this book by their encouragement, data, and criticism. To each of them, and especially to the following individuals, the writer wishes to express her debt of gratitude and her thanks: to staff members of the Psychiatric Divisions of Bellevue and Kings County Hospitals, and to the Bureau of Child Guidance of the New York City Board of Education, whose high quality of service is recognized throughout the country; the late Mayor F. H. LaGuardia of New York City, whose progressive mindedness and action in the field of social service have provided an example for civic leaders everywhere: Justices Justine W. Polier and W. Bruce Cobb; Edwin Lucas, Bernard Messenger, Emanuel Ebbin, Mrs. Catherine Alexander, Miss Florence Buckley, Mrs. Georgia Furst, Miss Rosetta Fisher, Miss Anna Heilmaier; and to her sisters, Mrs. Samuel Nemer, Mrs. Joseph Lichtenstein, and Miss Janet Goldberg. Special tribute is due to the late Dr. Caroline Zachry for her generous collaboration in organizing and developing the social service structure and policies of the School Part of the Children's Court of New York City.

Acknowledgment is also made of invaluable aid in the preparation of the manuscript by Miss Mary Bandayan. H. L. G.

CONTENTS

FOREWORD   vii

CHAPTER I   Children in Court   1

Truancy as a symptom, 1; Coordination of the efforts of courts, schools, and social agencies, an example, 4

CHAPTER II   Mentally Retarded Children   11

Groupings by psychometric and achievement tests, 11; Idiots, imbeciles, and morons, 17; Borderline and dull normal, 18; Cases, 19

CHAPTER III   Emotionally Unstable Children and Those with Neurotic Patterns   37

The mildly unstable child, cases, 37; The markedly unstable child, cases, 53; Neurotic patterns, 55, cases, 57

CHAPTER IV   Neurotics and Psychoneurotics   82

Neurotics, cases, 82; Deep anxiety, cases, 89; Schizoid features, 98, cases, 99; Psychoneurotic patterns, cases, 102

CHAPTER V   Psychopathic Personalities and the Mentally Ill   113

Psychopathic personalities, 113, cases, 115; The mentally ill, 123; Schizophrenia, dementia praecox, cases, 127; Manic-depressive psychosis, cases, 140; Possible brain disorders, cases, 143

CHAPTER VI	The Physically Ill and the Socially Handicapped	147

Physical illness, 147, cases, 148; The socially handicapped, 151, cases, 152; Placement needed, cases, 154; Placement not needed, cases, 169

CHAPTER VII	A Challenge to Community Organization	178

The problem, 178; Causal factors, 180; Diagnosis, 184; Treatment, 195; The role of the schools, 201; Children's courts, 210; Social agencies, 214

CHILD
OFFENDERS

CHAPTER I

CHILDREN IN COURT

ALMOST EVERYONE who speaks of juvenile delinquency has his own theory as to its meaning, how it is caused and what should be done about it. Even those to whom the term is applied occasionally refer to it in familiar tones. If the increased interest in child offenders can be focused upon the fundamental problems involved, substantial progress can be made, but all too frequently the response is merely, "Oh, you mean parent delinquency," or "All children are more or less bad." Often such statements are used as a springboard for one's own favorite concept of causality such as poverty, feeblemindedness, or broken homes.

Students of sociology and social work, teachers, social service personnel, and others deeply concerned about children who face court action desire definitive material on the subject. They realize what a catchall the expression juvenile delinquency has become, since it includes the most trivial misbehavior as well as arson, rape, burglary, and murder. Not only is every economic group represented but these children range from comparatively well integrated personalities to the untreatable of the mentally ill and from near genius to imbecile in intelligence.

This book is designed to help deepen our understanding of child offenders and their treatment. It seeks to portray the underlying behavior patterns of children whose first encounter with the law is truancy or misconduct in school. There is general agreement among social workers and allied groups that most criminal careers start with habitual truancy, although there is no implication that every truant becomes a criminal or that truancy produces criminality.

A promising field of investigation is thus offered, for if we can determine what causes persistent, unauthorized school absences and deal effectively with these factors, much delinquency could be prevented. At a critical period in their lives a substantial number of young people could be helped towards constructive paths. They and their parents could be spared tragic experiences. Communities would be protected from considerable aggression and loss while benefiting from a greater proportion of productive, useful citizens. Exploration of truancy is well worth attention and experiment.

Those who work directly with children in difficulties—social workers, probation officers, judges, psychologists, and psychiatrists—are forced to the conclusion from repetitions in daily practice that habitual truancy is symptomatic behavior. Just as varying pulse rates, temperatures, and blood counts are indicative of medical ailments requiring skilled diagnosis and care, so is persistent truancy an outward symbol of something amiss. School attendance, except for sickness or other valid excuse, is a child's daily responsibility, a vital part of his reality corresponding to an adult's regular presence at his job in factory, office, or shop. Every school session brings to all pupils constant problems of adjustment, of learning, of give and take with others. Its demands and pressures, presumably designed and geared to a child's needs and capacities, are similar in effect to those of a job or position in the adult world.

The boy or girl who constantly remains away from classes is fleeing from these responsibilities into a temporary freedom of loafing in the streets or at home, frequenting motion pictures, or allied activities. This escape from his reality denotes something or a constellation of things awry in his home, school, neighborhood, or within himself, causing an inability or unreadiness to cope with the exactions of school.

Truancy is thus a danger signal warranting full, timely inquiry and action. Experience demonstrates that the more fixed the pattern the harder it is to help the child. Yet repeatedly the problem goes unnoticed except by teachers who, with overcrowded classrooms and limitations in their own training, often remain unaware of its deeper significance. Recurringly, the child remains away most of a semester or two before anything is done.

At times schools are assailed for emphasizing attendance or are accused of being more concerned with a loss in state aid due to absentees than with the pupils. There is some truth in the latter as exemplified when principals urge attendance officers to place truants bodily in their classrooms. Upon the registers these pupils are marked present to prevent a diminution of state fiscal allotments. Many disappear from the school with the noon recess or on succeeding days and the reasons for their absence are not sought. After a number of such episodes, the principal might ask the truant officer to take punitive action against the child or his parents. On the other hand, there are principals whose attempts at a more enlightened program are hindered by lack of social and clinical facilities. Not until there is at least one skilled social worker functioning in each large school will truancy receive the skilled attention it needs.

Conflict among attendance officers and supervisors as to their goals reflects a sad social lag. Some continue to regard themselves as policemen whose role is to apprehend these children, scold them, and then escort them to school or court, with time out for berating the parents. Others believe their major function is to ascertain why a child is a truant and to try to alleviate the situation. Among the latter are those who have had social service training or who wish to acquire it. Analysis of court records indicates a preponderance of evidence in favor of the second group.

Great credit is due the late Dr. Caroline Zachry, who, as

Director of the Bureau of Child Guidance, New York City Board of Education, encouraged teachers and attendance officers to study mental hygiene principles and methods. She conducted outstanding training sessions throughout her brief tenure and was convinced that teachers and attendance personnel have excellent opportunities in the realm of prevention and treatment.

In our law, habitual truancy is classified as an act of juvenile delinquency, and children's courts have jurisdiction over truants, their parents and guardians. It is considered a lesser offense than theft, assault, etc., and practices, procedures, and methods within these courts reflect this view. When a truant is referred to court there is a tendency to feel that he does not need the study and care that those who are brought in for more serious misbehavior require. If the harassed court attaché, already overburdened by a multitude of cases, does not find evidence of an additional offense chargeable to the same child, such as theft, the matter generally receives scant attention.

Such emphasis upon the type of wrongdoing rather than upon the child seems to be a survival of a philosophy embedded in criminal law and penal codes where stress continues to be on the crime itself, not on the person charged with the transgression. In given instances, a truant may need the court's help far more than another offender who was led into a theft.

Many of the recidivists in children's courts for assault, burglary, rape, and homicide were first encountered there as truants. Query: Could their later misdeeds have been prevented if sufficient skill had been applied at their first court appearances, or within the educational system?

For more than a decade educators in New York City have been actively dissatisfied with the local children's courts. Lack of sufficient staff, together with a scarcity of clinical and placement resources and judges untrained in the psychology of childhood, accounts for some of this feeling. A timorous public relations policy has increased the difficulties these courts meet in attempting to fulfill their purposes.

Johnny, who stayed away from school sixty-two days out of ninety and menaced teachers and students with homemade guns and sharp-edged knives after stealing from lockers and the principal's office, was told by the judge to go home and be a good boy. The school authorities were disgusted and disheartened, unaware that the judge was helpless to do much else in this case, as no detention placement was available, no child guidance clinic could try to help John, as intake was closed due to staff shortages, and the family service agency counseling with John's parents could not gain access to him. What the principal and teachers realized was that Johnny was now bragging to his schoolmates that courts mean nothing, and his behavior was worse than before his appearance in court.

While public and private groups argue as to whether or not New York City or New York State should accept responsibility for furnishing the children's courts with a few rudimentary tools in the shape of additional clinical and placement opportunities, these incidents are multiplying throughout the metropolitan area. Few people know better than the delinquents themselves how impotent our children's courts are in dealing with a large number of them. That is why so many youthful offenders graduate into criminal courts on misdemeanor and felony charges. Unfortunately, the public is unaware of these grave conditions, and the courts by themselves cannot correct a condition which is wasteful in human lives and in money and tragic in its implications.

Similarly to children's courts in other regions, those in New York City have found themselves with a steadily mounting intake and graver charges were given precedence over others. In 1942 a temporary arrangement was made whereby they agreed to accept twenty-five referrals from the Bureau of Attendance each week. Strange as it may seem, that Bureau allocated five to each of its five divisions over the city, notwithstanding great diversity in density of population.

After handling cases of burglary and similar offenses, judges and other court workers did not deem it necessary to spend much time on truancy, especially as they were inclined to feel that attendance officers had not prepared their cases adequately or had not exhausted other methods of dealing with these children. It was also felt that the schools were to blame in not making classes more interesting. On the other hand, attendance officers felt their cases were rushed through the court and that they were not given sufficient opportunity to give the facts.

When the quota plan outlined proved unworkable as truancy and other school cases accumulated in large numbers, a new project was adopted under the sponsorship of the late Mayor F. H. LaGuardia. His profound sympathy for people in trouble and his sincere interest in children found expression in humane projects. With his encouragement, the Acting Presiding Justice of the Domestic Relations Court authorized the establishment of a special division in April 1944. Called the School Part of the Court, it has jurisdiction over such cases as truancy, unlawful detention of children from school by parents or guardians, and misconduct within schools. In place of the rotating system of judicial assignments in effect throughout other branches of the Court, one judge presides over this division.[1]

The purpose of the School Part is to seek fundamental causes of persistent truancy and to help these offenders sufficiently to prevent their becoming serious delinquents. To these ends, the Court has mobilized health, welfare, and educational services of public and private groups. From its inception, emphasis has been placed upon an integration of services for the benefit of children. With the help of the Superintendent of

[1] Since October 1946, an additional judge has been assigned to the School Part.

Schools, measures were taken to obtain qualified staff members and appropriate sites for hearings, which are informal and are held in school buildings, one for each county.

In the first two years of its existence, the School Part served approximately two thousand children as well as numerous parents and guardians. Moreover, firms and individuals charged with unlawful employment of minors, or with other acts contributing to their delinquency or neglect, were brought before the Court. Most of its referrals were received from the Bureau of Attendance, which is no longer restricted to a quota. The remainder comes from other divisions of the Domestic Relations Court and from social agencies. They concerned not children who played "hookey" for a day or two but those who had been absent for months, semesters, or years, although the Court itself placed no specific time limit. Although it felt that early truancy would be more amenable to treatment, it was recognized that many long-term cases had accumulated and required attention.

The office staff consists of six attendance officers, two part-time psychiatric social workers from the Bureau of Child Guidance, two policemen from the Juvenile Aid Bureau for special field investigations, a court reporter, an assistant court clerk for petitions and other legal process, a clerk, and two stenographers.

Functions in the School Part are divided into three phases: pre-judicial, judicial, and follow-up. As a case is received, it is registered and then studied individually to learn just what the problems are. In this sifting or screening process, attention is centered upon causal factors—what is producing the misbehavior. The second step is to determine how the difficulty can be corrected or eliminated. If this can be done without judicial process, no petition is taken, and an adjustment is attempted with the cooperation of the parents, their children, the school, health and welfare agencies.

Thus, where both parents were deeply troubled by the

wrongdoing of their young son who had had numerous accidents, including a brain concussion, and who spent most of his time riding subways, they were encouraged to obtain immediate medical and psychiatric care for him. Since then, he has shown considerable improvement. No court hearing was necessary as the parents were eager and ready to provide help. The Court considers its nonjudicial work as important as the judicial.

Cases are prepared for petition and hearing where it is plain that the court's power should be invoked for the wellbeing of children. At times a decision must be reached as to action against a person alleged to be contributing to the child's misbehavior. It is believed that effective proceedings in these instances are a vital step in the prevention of delinquency. Many of the firms and individuals involved have cooperated to the fullest extent once the issue has been made known to them. Since these hearings, a number of companies have evolved specific methods for preventing unlawful employment of minors in their establishments.

The Court's power to obtain needed medical attention is a potent force for benefiting children. Wherever possible this is done with the participation of the parents, but if they are lax and indifferent needed care is secured notwithstanding.

Informal hearings are scheduled as promptly as possible and all parties and interested persons are given full opportunity to express themselves so that the Court may get at the truth. On occasion it has been necessary to utilize warrants. An example of this was where a mother living apart from her husband was so mentally disturbed that she did not respond to summonses and insisted upon keeping her 9 year old son within their apartment at all times. She regarded him as a baby and would not allow him to attend school. As soon as they were brought in on a warrant, it was seen that both she and her boy needed hospitalization. They were sent to Bellevue under court order when voluntary help was refused, and there she was found to be psychotic. Her child's development had been so adversely affected by her behavior that he was almost at the stage of needing commitment to an institution for the mentally ill. With his father's aid, excellent care was obtained for him, and he has made marked progress.

Usually the case does not end with the hearing. In the child's interest, further work must be done to implement the judicial decision, which is not self-executing but offers a framework for social action. To this end, the resources of various educational, social, and health groups need mobilizing and their active sharing in the planning is desirable. Oftentimes school adjustments are essential, such as transfer to a different class, grade, or school. In many instances immediate medical service is imperative, such as care of the eyes, teeth, venereal treatment, tonsillectomies, or other surgery. Psychiatric care is needed for certain of these children or their parents; financial assistance or counseling may be required. After thorough study, if the home is found to be utterly destructive and the child should be removed for his own protection, the problem of finding a suitable placement arises.

A large number of these families are receiving aid from other agencies, public and private, and an integration of these services must be achieved for qualitative work. It is seen that the judicial decision is an invaluable element in a continuous process, for careful analysis and effort must precede it and additional planning and action must follow.

Records within a children's court are a treasure house of source material which should be used to help provide an authentic foundation for study and practice. All too often these files are neglected, although in them are to be found the tests of theories both as to causative factors and treatment. The cases that follow, each of which has been given a fictitious name to protect individuals' privacy, have been selected from records within the School Part.

Those who know the limitations of existing facilities and

the demands upon these will be cognizant of the persevering efforts with heart-breaking setbacks to obtain full clinical study in each and care for some of those needing substitute homes. All known causal factors are operative in these portrayals. They were chosen as representative of the total case load. An attempt has been made to fuse the existing social, medical, psychological, and psychiatric data so that each child discussed will emerge as an entity. Prognoses are given, not as final answers, but as an attempt to stimulate thought and discussion.

Social workers and judges are faced with the task of synthesizing information from these specialized fields of knowledge so that ignorance, prejudice, and whim can be replaced by skilled understanding gained through the utilization of expertness. Of necessity, legal, judicial, and administrative elements are also present as these may facilitate or block both study and treatment. To see each child as he really is and as a whole, to realize his particular needs and strengths is the first step in rehabilitation. Treatment which is not based upon accurate and full knowledge of the individual usually fails of its purpose. Experience teaches that the vast majority of youthful culprits can be helped to become law-abiding citizens. Our task is to help chart the way and not to remain dependent upon the method of trial and error.

CHAPTER II

MENTALLY RETARDED CHILDREN

To assist the reader in analyzing the cases presented in this and succeeding chapters, a brief outline of psychological groupings is given. Child offenders run the gamut from the intellectually gifted to imbecile, but often their educational achievement does not correspond to their innate capacity. Individual psychometric and achievement tests when given by experts in this field have important diagnostic value to social workers and judges in attempting to help delinquents.

To be valid, the scores obtained must be as accurate a gage as possible, with the examiner aware of accompanying circumstances: emotional blocking, fatigue, or other physical handicaps, and cultural background. For the nonpsychologist, any interpretation should be clear, forthright, and couched in nontechnical as well as technical terms. The name of the specific test, together with the score received, should be included because of variations among psychological examinations. Decisions as to a child's future are too vital to be based upon the results of group tests or those administered by persons with a smattering of training in mental measurements. Only those who have acquired special knowledge, skill, and clinical experience are in a position to know the pitfalls, the weaknesses, and the strengths inherent in the testing and interpretive processes. They are the ones who are qualified to test and to explain the results attained.

It is inevitable that a social worker's planning for a child of superior mentality will differ from that for a child of such low intelligence that he cannot do the work of the primary grades. This inevitability stems from the fact that these children's needs, other than for physical care and affection, differ and their capacities for utilizing various forms of help differ because of their varying mental abilities. Then again, planning for a child of normal mentality in the eighth grade who has not yet learned to read will differ from that for a child of the same age but of inferior intelligence who is a nonreader. So it goes, with each one's needs somewhat different from others of his age and sex. Thus an accurate knowledge of a child's intellectual capacity and achievement is essential in aiding him to function adequately.

Psychometric or psychological tests are devised to measure intelligence.[1] As has been pointed out,[2] the most widely used one is the 1937 Terman and Merrill revision of the Stanford-Binet. Originally the Stanford-Binet was used to discover the feeble-minded among French school children and was found to have a high correlation with actual scholastic achievement. Terman and Merrill modified and adjusted this test to the cultural and educational aspects of the United States. For greater reliability, they restandardized it and added another form for retesting. The L and M forms can be utilized interchangeably to guard against coaching. Note that the Stanford-Binet test was designed primarily for children and is not particularly useful in ascertaining high intelligence.

In the Terman-Merrill revision there are over 124 items arranged by years from a mental age of 2 to 14, together with tests at the average adult level and three levels of superior adult functioning. A child of normal intelligence who is not emotionally disturbed can answer almost all of the questions

[1] For a fuller discussion of tests and measurements, see Perry M. Lichtenstein and S. M. Small, *A Handbook of Psychiatry*. New York, W. W. Norton & Co., Inc., 1943, Chaps. IV and V.
[2] *Ibid.*, Chap. IV.

for his age. But emotional dysfunctioning can cause a wide deviation in scores, so that the final result will not approximate his innate ability but instead will reflect his present functioning capacity. That is why it is imperative that the examiner be alert to signs of dysfunctioning and record these.

The term I.Q., or intelligence quotient, is calculated as

$$\frac{\text{Mental age (determined by the test)}}{\text{Chronological age expressed as a percentage}}$$

For example, a child who scored a mental age of 5½ in the test and whose actual age is 10 years and 2 months has an I.Q. of 56. Terman and Merrill grouped intelligence levels as follows:

I.Q.	Classification
Below 70	Feeble-minded
70–80	Borderline deficiency
80–90	Dullness
90–110	Normal average intelligence
110–120	Superior
120–140	Very superior
Above 140	"Near" genius or genius

The Army Alpha and Beta examinations, utilized in both world wars, were designed as group tests to be administered to hundreds of persons at the same time instead of individually. For those who are almost illiterate or who know little English, the Beta form is used. As the names suggest, these are for adults rather than children.

Dr. David Wechsler of Bellevue Hospital formulated a psychometric test especially for adults which is known as the Bellevue-Wechsler examination, composed of ten parts.[3] He criticized Terman for stating that an I.Q. below 70 definitely shows feeble-mindedness. According to Dr. Wechsler, a definite

[3] David Wechsler, *The Measurement of Adult Intelligence*. Baltimore, Williams and Wilkins Co., 1939.

number cannot be set up as a dividing point between normal intelligence:

A mental defective is an individual who, when tested with a well-standardized intelligence examination, attains a score or rating which places him among the lowest two to three per cent of his age group with respect to the abilities measured, and with respect to such other abilities as may be deemed requisite for effective social adjustment. . . . A mental defective is not a person who suffers from a specific disease, but one whose general intellectual inadequacy allocates him to a social group whose level of functioning is such as to make it impossible for him to cope with his environment.

In short, according to Dr. Wechsler, one whose score is among the lowest 2 to 3 per cent of scores made by hundreds of others in his age group is feeble-minded. Within the Bellevue-Wechsler test are the following parts:

General Information, with questions in a wide range.
General Comprehension.
Arithmetical Reasoning, with problems of increasing complexity.
Ability to Repeat Digits, with numbers to be repeated forward or backward.
Detection of Similarities between two objects or concepts.
Picture Sequence, where the subject is allowed one to two minutes to arrange a series of pictures in sequence so that a story is told. A bonus in credits is given for speed.
Object Assembly where items are to be assembled in a given time. The time used fixes the credit received.
Block Design where the subject duplicates a varicolored design with a maximum time limit and special credit for speed.
Digit Symbols similar to item 4 of the Army Beta test where each digit is assigned a symbol and these are then filled in under a series of numbers. A vocabulary test is the alternative.

After the Bellevue-Wechsler examination has been taken, there are two ways of computing the results. The subject may be rated on the full scale, which comprises all of the ten tests mentioned above. Or the examiner may score the verbal tests (the first five items) separately from the performance tests (the last five items). The second rating method is preferred, for the person's verbal ability may differ markedly from his ability on performance tests and a better understanding of his specific capacities may be obtained. It has been found that the Bellevue-Wechsler scale is especially valuable in the testing of adolescents.

Psychometric examinations for the measurement of vocational interests [4] are also helpful in certain instances. These may aid in ascertaining special aptitudes, such as superior mathematical ability or manual dexterity.

Whatever the test, it is essential for the examiner to establish a satisfactory rapport with the subject, although it is recognized that this may not be possible where the person tested is in a highly disturbed state. There are cases in which children as well as adults were unable to complete the tests, not through lack of intelligence but because of emotional blockings. A skilled, experienced examiner is aware of these factors and records attitudes as well as scores for the guidance of social workers and judges who are trying to help the individual.

It has been found particularly valuable to have the Rorschach blot test given and interpreted together with the usual psychometric tests. Emotional deviations which may indicate the advisability of a psychiatric study either in a clinic or hospital often show up in the Rorschach pattern.

Mental deficiency and its synonyms, mental retardation and feeble-mindedness, have been defined as including all degrees of mental defect occasioned by arrested or imperfect mental development, as a result of which such a person cannot compete on equal terms with normal people nor can he manage himself or his affairs with ordinary prudence.[5]

[4] See Morris S. Viteles, *Industrial Psychology*. New York, W. W. Norton & Co., 1932.
[5] Perry M. Lichtenstein and S. M. Small, *A Handbook of Psychiatry*. New York, W. W. Norton & Co., Inc., 1943, p. 74. This is the definition accepted by the American Association on Mental Deficiency.

Psychometric tests constitute one method of discovering mental retardation in a child or adult and are valuable in determining the degree of feeble-mindedness in the individual. For accuracy in diagnosis, it is essential to consider his health, economic status, facilities for study, his social and developmental history. People who score below normal include two groups: (1) those who are congenitally feeble-minded, and (2) those whose mental processes have deteriorated due to mental illness, brain trauma, or an infectious or degenerative disease affecting the central nervous system.[6] In the second group are found some people who formerly functioned at a high intellectual level.

Although the term "congenitally feeble-minded" means those born mentally retarded, it also includes mental defectives up to five or six years of age. Glandular imbalance, congenital syphilis, or an infectious disorder in the mother may affect adversely the central nervous system of the fetus, producing mental retardation. Birth trauma, unsuccessful abortion, or brain hemorrhage at delivery may contribute toward the same result. Disease or disorder affecting the central nervous system up to about six years of age may impair the intellect to such a degree as to cause feeble-mindedness.

Five groupings are made of the mentally retarded: idiots, imbeciles, morons, borderline, and dull normal. The first are readily discernible. In the others examiners look for physical signs of degeneracy, particularly of the skull, eyes, nose, and palate. When the more obvious cases have been eliminated, suspected cases selected because of apparent clumsiness, lack of bodily equilibrium, blank, stupid facial expression, gross peculiarities of drawing, difficulties in reading and writing are given simple psychometric tests; borderline cases are given more intensive psychological study.

[6] *Ibid.*, 75 ff.

Idiots

On the Stanford-Binet test, the mental age of idiots is up to 3 years and their I.Q.'s range from 0 to 25. Those in the lower group cannot dress themselves, cannot talk so as to be understood, cannot develop habits of cleanliness; they need continuous attention. Those in the upper range can be taught a few habit patterns of cleanliness. Generally, idiots neither walk nor talk until late in life and then only to a limited extent. Some of them never walk or talk but just sit in one place swaying or motionless. Convulsions are frequent. Among idiots, lesions in the central nervous system are often found.

Imbeciles

Imbeciles have a mental age scale from 3 to 7 with I.Q.'s from 25 to 50. They can be taught to dress and wash themselves and do simple tasks. Those in the higher range can learn to protect themselves from obvious physical danger. Normal children learn to walk and talk earlier than imbeciles do.

Morons

On the Stanford-Binet test, morons attain a mental age of from 7 to 12 years, with I.Q.'s from 50 to 70. They have fewer physical stigmata (deformities and paralyses) than either idiots or imbeciles. Although not possessing ordinary judgment and the capacity to discriminate, they can do simple, routine tasks. Often the high-grade moron is successful as a porter, janitor, factory or road worker, in fact in any occupation which demands a minimum of mental effort. On the other hand, a low-grade moron needs a protective environment, for if it is not favorable, he makes an unsatisfactory life adjustment.

Many morons become useful, law-abiding residents in a peaceful social sphere. But as they are easily led and highly suggestible, those coming into the periphery of criminals or delinquents may readily become involved in misconduct. A number of the morons coming to the attention of children's courts and criminal courts have been the tools of more intelligent wrongdoers. Since a mental defective seldom considers the possible consequences of his actions and rarely has the capacity for self-restraint, it is not astonishing that he turns to crime, and his chances of rehabilitation are slim indeed.

Borderline

Those with I.Q.'s from 70 to 80 are the borderline group of mental defectives. To a large degree their social adjustment hinges upon the relative simplicity or complexity of their surroundings. In rural areas, in small urban centers, and in protected family situations even in metropolitan centers their chances of satisfactory adjustment are fairly good. Adequate supervision and training may help a potentially feeble-minded individual to become dull normal and function quite satisfactorily in society.

Dull Normal

Those with I.Q.'s from 80 to 90 are termed "dull normal." Even with disabilities in mathematics, abstract thinking, concepts, etc., they can manage independently in many fields of endeavor if they exert themselves to the utmost. When they are unwilling to try hard, they tend to become behavior problems at home, school, or on their jobs and often come into conflict with the law.

It has been recognized for decades that in given instances, mental deficiency may be a primary causal factor in misconduct,[7] and the cases which follow exemplify this principle. Where lack of normal intelligence is coupled with emotional disturbance, the results often border on the disastrous.

[7] J. McV. Hunt, ed. *Personality and Behavior Disorders.* New York, Ronald Press, 1944. Simon H. Tulchin, *Intelligence and Crime.* Chicago, University of Chicago Press, 1939.

MILDRED A.

Mildred, a heavy-set Negro girl of 15, in 8A grade, was referred to the School Part of Children's Court because of her serious misbehavior and excessive absence from school. In one outburst of temper she assaulted a fellow student and attempted to strike her with a large pair of shears. Mildred's language was vile and abusive, and she seemed to take pleasure in intimidating her classmates. After a long series of threatening acts towards teachers, Mildred attacked one by scratching her and tearing her clothing.

A check of social service exchange clearances and discussions disclosed that Mildred is the second illegitimate child of a mother who, while intoxicated, stabbed her paramour and served a prison sentence for manslaughter. At one time she suffered from a manic-depressive psychosis and was committed to a state hospital. She was imprisoned after having lived with various men, one of whom, Mr. E., took Mildred to reside with him. Mildred spent several years in orphan asylums. Her maternal aunt, a domestic, sometimes referred to as Mr. E.'s "girl friend," shares the same apartment. He is employed in the freight yards of a railroad company. He is friendly toward Mildred but is afraid of her temper tantrums.

While under the jurisdiction of the Court, Mildred was remanded to a temporary place of detention following an adjudication of delinquency. Her behavior there was so violent toward the other girls that she was transferred to Bellevue Hospital Psychiatric Division. While there she received full medical, psychological, and psychiatric study. The medical findings were negative. She rated borderline intelligence—an I.Q. of 74 on the Bellevue test: "There is sufficient inter and intra test variability to throw some doubt on the validity of the results. Test scores range from low defective to average levels, reflecting a high degree of emotional disturbance and instability. Educationally, she is over graded for her ability, and this may be a factor in her problem. Her arithmetic scores at 4A, with reading comprehension at 7A."

In the report of psychiatric observation, it was stated: "As you will note in the psychometric examination, Mildred's I.Q. is rather low, and it will be impossible for her to profit very much from academic schooling . . . her most disturbed behavior followed the death of her mother one year ago. . . . In view of Mildred's good adjustment during her stay in the hospital, it is recommended that she be given another opportunity on probation, but that she should receive psychotherapy and guidance. Also, all effort should be made to give her manual training rather than formal academic schooling."

The court then arranged for Mildred's transfer to a trade school and encouraged her to attend a psychiatric clinic. A referral was also made to a family service agency for counseling help. None of these efforts succeeded; Mildred's behavior continued to be explosive and abusive. She was unwilling to keep clinic appointments, and her truancy increased in severity. She was, therefore, committed to a correctional institution where she receives psychotherapy and supervision. From their report, she is showing slight progress. No noncorrectional placement was available for Mildred.

The reader will note that many elements mitigated against successful probation for Mildred. Her home conditions were irregular and unstable. Her habit of truancy was so well established that, lacking sufficient encouragement and satisfaction, it was much easier for her to continue with the old patterns while at home than to develop new ones. Such unfavorable home factors coupled with borderline intelligence do not provide a satisfactory basis for successful psychotherapy. The court recognizes that the prognosis for Mildred is poor. It is likely that she will engage in more serious delinquencies as she grows older.

JACK L.

Jack is almost 16 and is in the first year of high school. He was referred to the court because of chronic truancy. From his school record card it is clear that he has been truanting intermittently since he was in 1A. After two years in the first grade, he was enrolled in opportunity or ungraded classes until he was graduated from elementary school. During all this time he was marked D and unsatisfactory in scholastic achievement and personality traits. His teachers described him as insolent and lazy.

Jack's home life has been unhappy. His father died when Jack was an infant, and he was "boarded out" for three years as his mother worked long hours in a factory. She then remarried, but Jack has not liked his stepfather, and his two young half brothers' need for his mother's attention and care has not made it easier for Jack. Mr. L., the stepfather, has tried to reach Jack but without success, for he resists and feels Mr. L. is an interloper.

After a delinquency petition was taken, the court remanded Jack to Youth House, a place of temporary detention, for the purpose of a full study prior to a judicial decision regarding his future. Physically, Jack was found to need dental care, eyeglasses, and extra feedings. His nutrition was poor.

On the Wechsler-Bellevue scale, Jack scored an I.Q. of 77, indicating borderline intelligence. There was a marked scatter in the entire test pattern, which seemed to be due in part to Jack's severe educational retardation, as well as emotional conflicts which obscure a true picture of his intellective base. His fund of general information is scanty. Mental control and concentration are variable and barely adequate. In his responses Jack was very slow. On educational tests, his achievement in reading was nearer normal than his arithmetic score, which was exceedingly low. The psychologist concluded that his test responses suggested that his intellectual dysfunctioning may possibly be attributed to severe emotional factors. A marked speech defect is an additional handicap. Further academic instruction would be unproductive, but an indication of manipulative ability would warrant trade training at a simpler manual level.

In the psychiatric interviews Jack admitted thefts of toys from 5 and 10 cent stores and of money from roomers living in the same house. On one occasion he was detected, but the victim was a friend of the family and did not report the matter to the police. A few neurotic habits were revealed but no psychotic symptoms. Neurological examination was negative. Jack's adjustment at Youth House was fairly satisfactory. He tended to be seclusive. Although he did good work in shop classes, he was mischievous and careless. The psychiatrist concluded that more psychiatric interviews would be necessary to understand Jack's emotional problem. These were not possible at the time. No definite recommendation was given.

Since Jack was soon to reach 16, when he could receive an employment certificate, the court placed him on probation, not really expecting him to return to his academic classes for which he is so unprepared. But probation would help to assure compliance with the regulations governing the issuance of employment certificates and the obtaining of dental and other physical care. It was too late in the semester to arrange a transfer to vocational subjects.

In view of Jack's borderline intelligence and marked educational retardation, it is not at all surprising that he detests school. What a tragic waste it is that such boys are not taught simple trades in elementary school! To pass Jack from one grade to the next when he has not learned the work of the former and is woefully unprepared for the other, is as much an escape from reality as his truancy. This is not to say that a child should be forced to repeat the same grade indefinitely, for then similar problems are created. It should be better recognized that different children need different kinds of classes and schools. There could be elementary schools where the learning of manual skills replaces academic subjects for those who cannot learn academic subjects, and where a boy or girl could progress from one grade to another, for which he is given adequate preparation. From experience it appears that when classes are not geared to children's actual needs, truancy and misconduct are fostered and encouraged. It is no answer to reply that vocational schools exist, because these are mainly high schools, for admission to which standard elementary school graduation is required. Moreover, these high schools teach skilled trades which call for special aptitudes and an intelligence level above borderline. They, therefore, tend to exclude children like Jack who could not fit into their programs and who, therefore, need special facilities in the elementary school years.

BASIL B.

Basil, 13 years old and in the sixth grade, was referred to the School Part of Children's Court by the Bureau of Attendance for persistent truancy during the past three years. Analysis indicated that the case was one of chronic parental neglect, and therefore a neglect petition was taken. The marital relationship has never been good, and the parents have been separated for more than five years. When Basil was 9, his father was hospitalized for a year in a state institution for the mentally ill with the diagnosis "syphilis of the central nervous system." Prior to their separation, the parents quarreled constantly, with Mr. B. hurling abuses at Mrs. B. Both seem to lack interest in their children—Basil, his two older sisters, and a younger sister. For six years the family has been receiving public assistance. Mrs. B. is harassed and discouraged. Not being planful nor a careful buyer, she has hardship in managing on a relief allowance. She tries hard to keep the apartment clean and tidy.

Mrs. B. feels that Basil is beyond her control. He remains out late at night, refuses to go to bed until long past midnight, quarrels almost daily with Joan, the eldest sibling, who is 16. He will not get up to go to school, and the attendance officer reports that whenever he visits the home he finds Basil in bed. A year ago he was referred to a mental hygiene clinic, but he never returned for treatment. He was found by the examiners to be of dull normal intelligence with an I.Q. of 84; general personality difficulties were noted.

Basil was brought to the court's clinic for study upon an order by the judge. Medical findings were negative. Physically, Basil is well developed and free from defects. On the Stanford-Binet test his I.Q. was 85. His arithmetic is at the fourth-grade level, but in mechanical tests he is average. In the examiner's opinion Basil is considered to be operating at a low average level of intelligence. In psychiatric interviews of Mrs. B. and Basil, she was observed to be a high-strung, tense, hasty, and incompetent parent. He was seen to have good possibilities if his interests, energies, and outlooks were geared along socially desirable lines. Unfortunately, however, he has deviated from his duties and responsibilities into a world of dreaming and indolence and resorts to rationalizations and excuses in self-defense. He lacks insight and will become an increasingly grave social problem if his present patterns continue, perhaps a permanent misfit, even if not a criminal. He admitted losing a drugstore job because of instability, drifting into movies when he should have been on duty.

The clinic thereupon recommended placement of Basil in an institution for normal children to give him opportunities to develop new interests and new habits in a controlled environment. In vain, personnel of the court sought a placement for Basil. He was too old, too young, too retarded scholastically, not a disturbed enough personality, etc., for the very few openings available in private institutions, and there is no public institution for these children in the whole five boroughs of New York City.

The court had no alternative but to permit Basil to remain at home. From current reports his misconduct is becoming more severe while the court stands powerless to help him. Probation is ineffective here because of the inadequate home conditions. When will society awake to the fact that by failing to provide children's courts with proper tools, it stimulates the growth of juvenile delinquency and crime?

FRED W.

Fred, 14, and his mother, a part-time domestic worker, have made their home with her brother, Mr. S., since Mr. W. deserted the family eight years ago after a series of violent altercations. Mr. S. is separated from his wife, but his two children reside with him. Since his apartment is small, they are overcrowded, and Fred has been sharing a bed with his mother. She reported to the school guidance clinic where Fred was referred for testing a year ago that she has had great difficulty with him for a long time. He sets fires with papers. He steals and has an uncontrollable temper. At one time he was in court after he, with other boys, had opened a letter box in an apartment house. As a result he had been remanded to a shelter for two days and placed on probation for three months.

A report from the principal to an attendance supervisor outlines the problem: Because of his feeble-mindedness, Fred has become involved in all sorts of trouble. The social worker of the Department for Children of Retarded Mental Development (in one of whose classes Fred was a pupil) had been attempting to place him in an institution for some time, but has been unsuccessful. Although he has been fifteen terms in elementary school, he is unable to do work above the second-grade level. He is large sized but infantile in behavior. He is easily led and influenced by other children who make him the scapegoat of their pranks.

It is interesting to note the findings made by the Bureau of Child Guidance, to which Fred had been sent by the principal when it was obvious that he did not fit into his school. Thirteen years old at the time, he was found to be physically overmature for his age. Symptoms of an organic heart disease were present. There were signs of intellectual deterioration, with an I.Q. of 60 on the revised Stanford-Binet test. His reading and arithmetic scores were at the 2B level. In the preliminary psychiatric interview his instability was evidenced. The conclusion was reached that little could be done for Fred in his home environment and that his supervision and training were entirely inadequate. "Fred will undoubtedly become more and more maladjusted socially and his delinquency will probably increase. . . . It is urgent that he be placed in a state school for mental defectives." The clinic thereupon made an appointment for study in Bellevue Outpatient Mental Hygiene Clinic, hoping that Fred's mother would be willing to have him committed on a voluntary basis without the necessity for court action.

Accordingly, Fred was examined at the Bellevue clinic. No pathology was found in the physical and neurological examinations. On psychometric study his I.Q. was found to be 59. Psychiatric observation showed that Fred is highly suggestible, immature, and inadequate. His reasoning, insight, and judgment are defective. He is restless, aggressive, willful, and stubborn. The examiners concluded that he is a mental defective of moron level and advised his mother to consent to a commitment. She felt Fred would always blame her if she consented, so she refused, and the clinic then closed its case.

When all the data were received and reviewed by the court, it was decided to proceed on the truancy charge with an involuntary commitment through Bellevue Hospital Psychiatric Division, and a remand was ordered. Because ward observation and tests confirmed the diagnosis of mental defectiveness and his inability to adjust in the community, Bellevue Psychiatric Division applied for Fred's certification to a state school and he was committed there.

This case illustrates the need for authoritative handling of the commitment issue. Waiting for voluntary action by parent or guardian produces delay and in the interval the child may become linked with the most serious delinquency. Especially is this true where adequate supervision is lacking. Naturally, a parent or guardian, no matter how difficult the child's behavior, hesitates, postpones, and finally refuses consent in the vast majority of commitment cases. Not only do they fear being blamed by the child for "putting him away," but other relatives, including siblings, are also inclined to cast aspersions. Feelings of guilt are bound to come to the fore. Then again, in voluntary commitments release is usually easier, and the parent or guardian is continually torn by the feeling that if he desires it the child can be released. The court itself should assume and accept responsibility in these cases, making certain of course that a firm foundation for commitment exists in the particular case.

BRYAN C.

Bryan, almost 16 and in 8B grade, is the only child of divorced parents who have both remarried. Although he was given into the custody of his mother, Bryan has lived nearly all his life with his maternal grandparents. Bryan refused to attend school, contending that he is too big and should be allowed to work. When in class he was disobedient and insolent. When he threatened to punch his teacher and was told to report to the principal, Bryan walked out of school and refused to return, whereupon he was referred to the court for truancy. His companions were older boys with whom he spent much time on the streets.

In an effort to help Bryan, the judge ordered medical, psychometric, and psychiatric study in the court clinic. Bryan was found to be in fine physical condition with the height and weight of a 17 year old boy. He graded as dull normal in the Terman tests, with an I.Q. of 80. His reactions were very slow and showed uniform mental retardation. During the psychiatric examination Bryan was quiet in manner, withdrawn, had very little to say of his own accord, and comparatively little in response to encouragement and explanations. Without expressing it verbally, his attitude was one of mild resentment, feeling that the examinations and the court procedures were for the purpose of trying to make him do something which he did not want to do. He found it difficult to adjust himself to any disturbance of his immediate comfort, and exhibited a shallow egocentric childishness out of keeping with his years and general development. There was petulance, resentment, irritability, and a disinclination to attempt any planning.

Bryan thought the problem of attending school an uncomfortable one and he did not promise to attend school even for the few months until his sixteenth birthday when he could be excused. He spoke of three desertions from his home, two last year to Pennsylvania, and a third this year when he went to Florida with a friend who paid his way. In the latter state he was arrested as a vagrant, but his mother sent railway fare and he was released. Although Bryan did not admit that his parents' divorce and remarriages weighed on his mind, he gave an impression that these are painful subjects which he forced himself to avoid in discussion. He indicated that he is happiest with a group of older boys who accept him at his own value, whereas other people do not accept him as he is but demand intelligent consideration of situations and some foresight in dealing with these.

In the psychiatrist's opinion, Bryan has been handicapped not only by family instability but by intellectual dullness, which is responsible for many acts of poor judgment and his inability to view circumstances adequately. His problem is one of character development, and he might be helped by the program of a quasi-military school where he could receive training in personal responsibility and trade training.

No placement was available for Bryan so he continued as he had been doing until he reached 16; then he obtained a job as a stock boy and was granted an employment certificate by the educational authorities.

Bryan came to the court's attention too late for the court to be able to help him. He should have been referred there years ago. It is likely that his work record will be poor and he will drift from one unskilled job to another with intervals of unemployment.

JAMES C.

James is 12 years of age, small and thin. He has been in an ungraded class for the past three years. His family has been receiving public assistance for thirteen years, as Mr. C. is unemployable due to a cardiac condition and epilepsy. Mrs. C. is of low intelligence and a poor housekeeper, so that the home is untidy and dirty. Her sister is an inmate of a state school for the feeble-minded. Both Mr. and Mrs. C. are lax in supervising James and are careless about his school attendance. During the last two semesters James has been present sixteen days. He repeated each grade until his placement in the ungraded group. Feeling considerable pressure to earn money, James has been unlawfully employed by a truck driver delivering oil and ice. His employer exploits James by requiring long hours of work in return for a meager wage which looms large to James.

When he is in school James is disobedient, quarrelsome with his classmates, and defiant. He disrupts teaching sessions and games and is disliked by other children. Teachers reported him to their principal, and he in return urged the Bureau of Attendance to take James into court for truancy and misconduct. This was done, and the court was called upon to see what help could be obtained for James. Since it appeared that he might be mentally defective, he was remanded to Bellevue Hospital Psychiatric Division for a period of observation.

There James was given physical, neurological, and psychological examinations, and he was also observed by two psychiatrists. He was found to be an imbecile needing care in a state school for mental defectives and was committed to the same institution in which his maternal aunt is a patient.

James is so suggestible that it is a wonder he was not led into serious wrongdoing by older delinquents. If his truancy had continued much longer, this would undoubtedly have occurred. Ordinary schools require more of such an individual than he possibly can achieve, so it is not to be wondered at that he avoids school as much as possible.

WILL A.

Will, 14, is thin and undersized. Two of his older brothers are in state institutions for mental defectives, and the third is serving a prison term for burglary. There is deep-seated friction between his parents, who quarrel incessantly. On three occasions his father has been in Magistrates Court for disorderly conduct. One such appearance resulted from his tearing his wife's dress off her and beating her into unconsciousness. He is also known to Special Sessions Court for stealing a car. Both parents are hostile toward school and think it is clever of Will to fool the teachers by truanting and then making up excuses.

Mrs. A. is a poor housekeeper; consequently the home is dirty and a place the whole family avoids. Will spends most of his time roaming the streets in company with older boys who are known delinquents.

When Will was brought into Children's Court on a truancy charge, he revealed in discussions that he dislikes his parents and his home. He shows his resentment by truanting and frequent episodes of running away from home. Four times Will has been excluded from school for pediculosis. He is emotionally disturbed and nervous. Clinical study shows that he has an I.Q. of 64 and is retarded scholastically twelve terms. He needs placement, but no placement is available for him.

Will's home is so unstable and destructive that undoubtedly his present disturbance will increase, not diminish. With the lack of a suitable substitute home, it is likely that he will become more delinquent.

ARTHUR W.

Arthur is 15 and well grown. He came to the court's attention because of habitual truancy and late hours. Check of social service exchange data showed that both his parents are feeble-minded and alcoholic. His two sisters have been placed in institutions for sex delinquents. Arthur has run away from home eight times and expressed feelings of hatred toward his home and family. He has repeated each grade at least once, and some twice. With the physique of a man, he is in 5B with much younger and smaller children. He can't comprehend the lessons and feels horribly out of place in the classroom.

The court made arrangements for hospital study of Arthur. There it was found that he is a mental defective of moron level, with an I.Q. of 59 on the Bellevue intelligence test. During his stay in the hospital he was a severe disciplinary problem, was restless, quarrelsome, obscene and uncooperative. Medical examination was negative. The hospital made application for his commitment to a state school for mental defectives, and, despite the protests of his mother and uncle, he was ordered committed after a hearing in Supreme Court.

The question might well be asked: Why did not the school authorities deal with Arthur more effectively? His marked mental and scholastic retardation could and should have been discovered long ago. Why try to teach him subjects which are beyond his capacity to grasp? It is to his detriment and that of his fellow students and teachers to keep evading this issue. With modern testing methods and skills, the feeble-minded can be located well within the primary grades and provision for their care should be made then so as to obviate later school and personal difficulties.

EDWARD C.

Edward is 15½ years of age and has the physique of a man. He came into court on a charge of persistent truancy. From before Edward's birth his father has been at sea except for brief intervals, first in the maritime service, and then in the Navy. Mrs. C. is employed in a neighborhood tavern from 6 P.M. to midnight. Her friend, Mrs. M., lives with the family and acts as housekeeper. She complained to the Red Cross over a year previously that Edward was disobedient, uncontrollable, and destroyed his clothing. They referred the family to a private family agency for help but when appointments were not kept the case was closed.

Edward's school record denotes severe retardation and health problems, such as crossed eyes, poor muscle coordination, undue restlessness, and twitching movements. He refuses to do any assignments, shouts, is insolent and insubordinate. Frequently he runs out of the school building while classes are in session.

Under these circumstances the court felt that a period of observation at Bellevue Hospital Psychiatric Division would prove helpful, especially on the issue of mental deficiency. Their report is illuminating. The physical and neurological examination showed that Edward has scars on his right arm and right foot and an amputation of three toes of the right foot resulting from an electrocution which he suffered two years previously. He has certain neurological symptoms, such as irregular pupils, divergent squint, fluttering of closed eye lids, and convergence of outstretched arms. An electro-encephalogram (measurement of the brain waves) revealed some of the characteristics of idiopathic epilepsy. X-ray of the skull showed no fracture. Blood Wassermann test was negative. Eyeglasses are needed. An attempt at surgery was made to correct his crossed eyes (strabismus), but Edward became very disturbed when taken to the operating room and would not permit the operation.

He was found to function on a mentally defective level. On the Bellevue intelligence test he scored an I.Q. of 69. He is able to do third-grade reading and spelling, and fourth-grade arithmetic. During his stay in the hospital he was restless, overactive, overtalkative, and quarrelsome. He admitted stealing and truancy. In the examiners' opinion Edward has certain symptoms suggestive of organic brain disease, and eventually he will have to be committed to a state hospital for the mentally ill unless there is some change in his condition. Their report was summarized thus, "... it is our feeling that this boy is functioning as a mental defective at this time and that he has organic disease of the brain. We feel that placement in a state school (for mental defectives) is preferable now to commitment in a state hospital so that he may receive some further schooling. On —— day we made application for the boy's commitment to Wasaic State School. The mother did not appear to protest. The boy was committed to that institution and was transferred there on —— day."

The advisability of the Court's order of hospitalization was demonstrated by the medical and psychiatric findings. For his own protection and that of the community, Edward is better off at Wasaic than at home.

CHARLES W.

Charles, a 9 year old Puerto Rican boy, was referred to the School Part of Children's Court by a judge presiding over another branch of the Court. Mrs. W. had complained to the Bureau of Adjustment in Children's Court that he is ungovernable, beyond her control, refused to attend school, would not eat his meals, and roamed the streets until midnight. Believing he was "Superman," he jumped off a fire escape several months ago and broke an arm. He has made threats of self-injury and recently insisted that he will jump into the Harlem River. Periodically he has nightmares during which his mother is forced to wake him. He told her that sometimes in his dreams he returns home to find only her eye in the ashes of their house. He suffers from chronic insomnia and enuresis. From the start of his school career three years ago he has remained in 1A grade and has not learned to write his name. From the time Charles was an infant his parents have been separated, but he sees his father once each week. Mr. W. contributes twelve dollars weekly toward his son's support; Mrs. W. supplements this income by working as a garment operator. Four months prior to Charles' birth a sister, seven months old, died of a brain tumor. Two previous outpatient clinical examinations indicated Charles has borderline intelligence. His mother is a gaunt, nervous woman who appears as much in need of help as Charles.

The School Part sought the advice of Bellevue Hospital Psychiatric Division in planning for Charles. Psychometric tests showed that Charles has dull normal intelligence, I.Q. 83, and although educable, has no knowledge of reading, writing, arithmetic, or spelling. In psychiatric interviews he was observed to have poor social orientation. The examiners concluded that Charles is a deprived child who has suffered from his underprivileged status, poor cultural background, inadequate contact with English-speaking people, and insufficient home life, and shows some neurotic traits, but is not mentally defective. They recommended that Charles be placed in an institution for normal boys.

Although strong efforts were made to carry out this recommendation, it was impossible to do so because of overcrowded and insufficient private facilities and an utter lack of public placement opportunities for children such as Charles. One month later a report was received from Bellevue Hospital to the effect that Charles was returned there on transfer from another hospital where his mother was a patient. She had taken him with her as she had no place to leave him. In the absence of any other available placement, Charles was committed through Bellevue Hospital to a state school for mental defectives.

This case portrays a shocking condition. That a child of normal, though dull, intelligence should have to be placed with idiots, imbeciles, and other mental defectives because a great city such as New York fails to provide public facilities for his care, is an indictment of those who continue to oppose public child-care programs in favor of a policy of exclusive public subsidies to private institutions. It is understandable that private groups with limited facilities and budgets develop eligibility requirements of age, grade, sex, religion, physical condition, intelligence level, and personality adjustment. It is likewise understandable that they would prefer not to admit a child so scholastically retarded as Charles. If his case were the only one of its kind, there might be some excuse for the perpetuation of such an outmoded system. The tragedy is that his situation is typical of many hundreds of such cases, differing in one or more minute elements but basically similar.

There is great need for both private and public institutions and foster homes for children who cannot be helped sufficiently at home or with family members. Operation of well run public institutions for those children who for one reason or another are ineligible for admission to private institutions does not mean the elimination of the latter. In fact, they would be encouraged to blaze new trails in child care, since they would be relieved of the obligation of accepting some who do not fit into their already developed programs. An analogy can be drawn with the growth of public assistance systems which have freed private family agencies from the burden of long-time maintenance cases, thus enabling them to make innovations and concentrations of service which were not hitherto possible. Social workers and judges do not view this matter with complacency. They are trying vigorously to bring about a change, but until the public is sufficiently aware of the problem, their efforts will not succeed.

Another social lag reflected here is that Charles had to be labeled a delinquent child in order for the court to try to assist him. Under the Domestic Relations Court Act of the City of New York, like other acts governing children's courts, jurisdiction is limited to children who are charged with being delinquent, neglected, or dependent. Obviously, Charles could not be classified as neglected or dependent, since his mother was giving him reasonable care and he was being supported by both parents. Therefore, for the court to act there had to be a petition of delinquency against a 9 year old boy who was much more sinned against than sinning. Other examples of such rigidity in a law designed to protect children are found in the chapters that follow. More flexible practice should be possible in the interest of helpless children.

HELEN R.

Helen appeared in Children's Court because of habitual truancy. She is an attractive blonde of 15, large for her age and in 6B grade. Her school card indicates that she repeated 1A, 3A, 4B (twice), and 6A, and has had excessive absences for the past two years. Helen has an older brother, John, who had been studying to be a minister, an older sister, Gertrude, who is employed and three younger brothers. Helen does not get along well with her parents or her siblings, among whom there is considerable rivalry. Both John and Mrs. R. are fearful that Helen "will get into trouble; she does not learn what is right and what is wrong."

Last year her mother complained to a different branch of the court that Helen was beyond control, incorrigible, a truant, associating with very undesirable companions, stealing money from members of the family, and on one occasion remained away from home all night. At the court's request she was examined at the Mental Hygiene Clinic of Kings County Hospital.

Their report disclosed that psychological study was unsuccessful due to personality problems. In the psychiatric interview Helen was described as sullen, resentful, and untruthful. She was very protective in regard to her behavior and tended to blame her sister for difficulties at home. It was evident that she has been attempting a sophisticated social and sexual adjustment beyond her age and resents any supervision or advice from either parents or siblings. The classification made was "behavior problem with psychopathic personality traits." In the examiner's opinion, she is not amenable to guidance or probationary supervision in the home; if she remains in the community she will be a sex problem as well as a family problem; and she will not profit from academic instruction but should receive training along domestic lines or in a simple, unskilled trade. Because of a need for close supervision, commitment to a state correctional institution was recommended. The judge presiding over the case at that time decided not to follow this recommendation. After a week's remand to the S.P.C.C., a place of temporary detention, the case was closed.

When the available data were studied in the School Part, it became evident that a period of observation in Bellevue Psychiatric Division would be advisable, as the question of possible mental deficiency needed careful evaluation. Accordingly, a request for such a remand was made and granted by the presiding judge. Psychometric findings were as follows: On the Bellevue-Wechsler scale Helen earned a composite I.Q. of 61, testing about the same on the verbal and performance material. Functioning is somewhat uneven. General information is very poor. Comprehension and reasoning ability are relatively fair. Ability to manipulate number concepts is very poor. School achievement tests show Helen's accomplishments in reading and spelling to be at the 3B-4A level and in arithmetic barely at the 3A level, which is at least about one year below that expected of a girl of her mental status. She classifies as a mental defective of the high-grade moron to borderline level. Medical findings were negative, except for vaginal introitus.

Psychiatric observation on the ward indicated that Helen has the personality of an unstable delinquent girl. She expressed no feelings of either shame or guilt about her misconduct. On the contrary, her attitude is that she has been unjustly accused and mistreated. This is not a superficial attitude but a true belief on her part. Both psychiatrists and the psychologist strongly recommended that Helen be committed to a state school for the mentally retarded.

When this was discussed with Helen's mother and brother John, they objected vehemently and begged that Helen be given another opportunity at home. Although further delay was opposed by the social service staff of the court, the judge decided not to commit Helen as recommended on the ground that the psychologist described her as a high-grade moron. It was the judge's feeling that a high-grade moron should be able to get along in the community and does not need care in an institution.

Several months later the mother and John came to the judge and told him that they had been wrong in opposing commitment as Helen's misbehavior is more serious than before. She now consorts with members of the armed forces whom she encounters on the streets late at night. They despair of her health and her morals. But the judge remained unconvinced.

It would appear that the judge's own conceptions ran contrary to those of social workers, psychiatrists, and psychologists and that he preferred his own to theirs. If an institutional placement other than a state school for the mentally deficient had been available for Helen, he probably would have ordered a commitment. But in the face of the hospital findings no other placement was possible at the time. If the psychological findings had been worded differently, the judicial decision probably would have implemented them. It is likely that at a later hearing when Helen's misconduct becomes even more serious, the commitment recommended will be made.

CHAPTER III

EMOTIONALLY UNSTABLE CHILDREN AND THOSE WITH NEUROTIC PATTERNS

A VARIETY of emotional deviations are manifested in some of the children who appear in Children's Court. All gradations are represented, from slight nervousness and tension to mental illness and organic brain disorders. Starting with instances of mild instability, the illustrations presented in this and the following two chapters may serve to point out the diversity found.

THE MILDLY UNSTABLE CHILD

CLYDE S.

Clyde, 8 years old, is the only child of Mr. and Mrs. S., who separated when Clyde was six. He was referred to the court because of excessive school absences and fighting with other children when he attended his 2A class. His teachers described him as sullen, withdrawn, lacking friends, and clinging to his mother, with whom at times he is in open conflict when she is responsible for his tardiness. He sometimes came to school in a filthy condition and without underwear. A speech defect and general nervousness were noted on his school record card. The attendance officer and visiting teacher reported that Mrs. S. and Clyde lived in a messy furnished room and that they sleep together in a single bed. Neighbors have reported that she remains out until very late hours, keeping Clyde with her. The family was known to a social service agency where Mrs. S. had sought aid during two periods of separation. She expressed the hope that her husband would return each time and, therefore, failed to press for payment of his irregular contributions toward support. Mrs. S. was described by this agency as a generally disorganized individual of apparent dull mentality with nervous, uncontrolled tremors.

Both parents were interviewed by the court social worker, following which a neglect petition was taken as placement was indicated. Mr. S. related that he had known his wife for one year prior to their marriage. He had completed high school at night while employed on WPA and later by a trucking company. For the past three years he has been working as a laborer for the Navy, earning $35 weekly. He told the worker that there was constant quarreling, due to Mrs. S.'s neglect of the home, her failure to prepare meals, and her neglect of Clyde. Mr. S. added that he is at a loss to know what to do about Clyde; living with Mrs. S. is not good for the boy, but he, Mr. S., has no place for Clyde as Mrs. S. senior has been a patient in a state mental hospital for the past two years.

In interviews Mrs. S.'s disorganization and inability to care for Clyde were clearly evidenced. She repeatedly referred to him as a baby and expressed a need to cling to him, often keeping him home from school to be company for her. They would sleep until noon; then she would give him coffee and cake and take him out shopping all afternoon, accompanying him to her mother's house for supper and the evening, returning about midnight. While recognizing that such a program is not suitable for a child, she found herself doing this frequently. Sharing the apartment of her aged parents are three sisters whose husbands are in military service.

To assist the court in planning adequately for Clyde, the judge ordered medical, psychological, and psychiatric examinations for Mr. and Mrs. S. and Clyde, to be performed in the court's clinic. Mr. S. was found to be a well developed, sturdy man in good physical condition, except for impaired vision. On psychometric tests he achieved an I.Q. of 118, revealing elements of superior intelligence. In psychiatric interviews he was observed to be highly tense, irascible, impatient and self-opinionated. He displayed no trace of sympathy or regard for his wife's predicament and interprets the entire situation from his personal viewpoint of how he has been wronged and aggrieved by the marital failure. All blame he projects upon her. He complained that she has no mind of her own and is entirely guided, dominated and influenced by her parents, on whom she depends for everything but maintenance. Mr. S. has no affectionate feeling toward his wife and plans to divorce her. He made a random request that Clyde be placed in his custody, although he admitted that he has no facilities for Clyde's care and supervision. It was difficult for the psychiatrist to determine Mr. S.'s true feelings and thoughts toward Clyde, but it was obvious that there were no prospects for a reconciliation with Mrs. S.

In the medical report Mrs. S. is described as obese, well developed, and well nourished, with a possible pituitary disorder, and with nervousness reflected in a tic of the head which becomes prominent when she is under tension and in tremors of the fingers. On psychological tests she obtained an I.Q. of 79 which the examiner considered not to be fully representative. She succeeded at a higher level with tests involving matter of fact and arithmetic reasoning. Her sustained attention was poor and may account for the lowering of her rating. She is functioning at the dull normal level of intelligence, although her native capacity appears to be substantially higher.

Deviations were found on the psychiatric examination. She showed marked nervousness and confusion as to values and plans. With this she nevertheless maintains an atmosphere of composure and control, probably deriving from her obesity without which she very likely would be much more disorganized mentally. Although it was not possible to establish any signs of paranoid delusions or hallucinations, there was a suggestion of hypomanic coloring to her speech and reactions. The diagnosis made for her was "severe nervousness with vague borderline psychotic elements." The examiner was of the opinion that Mrs. S. would become thoroughly disorganized if Clyde were taken from her at this time, and therefore recommended that she be allowed to retain custody for the present. He also advised that she be rechecked in three to six months.

Clyde physically is well developed and well nourished, but needs glasses. He scored an I.Q. of 110 while showing retardation in school skills. He has high average intelligence but is not functioning at his best because of emotional factors. In psychiatric interviews he was seen as pleasant, friendly, cooperative and well meaning, with some insecurity and timidity reflected in his manner due to the oversolicitude of his mother, who continually hovered over him. The examiner believed that Clyde's nervous restlessness may be a factor in his maladjustment at school. Lack of parental discipline was also evinced in his behavior. He was diagnosed as a mildly unstable boy for whom placement would be desirable. Inasmuch as his mother vehemently opposed placement and was on the verge of a complete breakdown, delay was counseled for her sake. It was concluded that Clyde exhibited no vicious traits and that his mild instability was due to situational circumstances.

The court realized that a substitute home would have to be found for Clyde in his own best interests, even though the psychiatrist's recommendation was accepted for the time being. Therefore, placement avenues were explored in the expectation that Clyde's home conditions would soon become unbearable and a suitable substitute home is sometimes impossible to find. Two months later Mrs. S. literally dragged Clyde into the clinic and evidenced such marked mental deterioration that the psychiatrist urged the court to place Clyde immediately. Her behavior was recognized to be extremely harmful to his health and welfare.

Strenuous efforts were made by the court to effect a placement for Clyde with normal children of his age group. No such public facilities exist in the City of New York, and the only private agency which had an opening at first insisted that parental consent be obtained as a prerequisite to admission. While it is realized among social workers and others that parental consent is highly desirable and much preferable to a compulsory placement in increasing the likelihood that it will be successful for the child and his parents, it was futile to expect either Mr. S. or Mrs. S. to consent. The court had tried to secure their consent, but Mr. S. was unwilling and unable to assume responsibility; he still talked vaguely of planning to request his mother's release from a mental institution so that she could make a home for Clyde. Mrs. S. was too disturbed emotionally to consider her son's welfare above her uncontrollable impulses. When the court persisted and emphasized to the agency that Clyde was in grave danger of developing serious personality difficulties were he to remain with his mother, he was admitted on a four months' remand.

Just prior to the expiration of the remand, a very interesting report of Clyde's progress was sent to the court by the institution. It is worth while to set forth the contents in some detail:

"During the first two months Clyde was under care, he was handicapped in becoming accustomed to his new life because he was so immature and unprepared to assume any responsibility for himself; he made no friends, could not adjust to the cottage routine by doing his share of chores or being reasonably able to care for his physical welfare. However . . . [afterwards] there was definite improvement . . . as evidenced by his greater ability to care for himself physically, to cooperate in doing chores and to be accepted by his contemporaries. This development has been gratifying to Clyde, who feels quite contented at [the institution], though he would prefer to live with his family.

"Clyde has attended school regularly and has shown an increasing interest in his studies. He was very restless at first, but he is now more able to concentrate. Despite his good intelligence (I.Q. 113) his progress has been slow, yet he was promoted to 3A because of his real effort and improved achievement. Since he was practically a nonreader on admission, we arranged to give him remedial instruction. A recent test after two months of this special help reveals that he has gained a year in reading ability. He is very pleased with his school progress.

"Our psychiatric study of Clyde disclosed that he was an unstable, emotionally immature boy who was definitely affected by the unwholesome relationship to his mentally disturbed mother. Our psychiatrist believed that it would be to Clyde's welfare if we tried to help him to a better understanding of his mother and encouraged a closer contact with his father. Further psychiatric treatment may be indicated should the boy remain under our care.

"Throughout this period Clyde has been visited almost weekly by his father, while his mother visited only intermittently, stating that she did not receive the necessary funds from the father to come more frequently. Although both parents met occasionally at [the institution] they did not let their personal disagreements cause unhappiness to Clyde. During Christmas vacation the boy lived with his maternal grandparents, an arrangement worked out by Mr. S. at our suggestion, but saw his parents separately. Clyde still feels closer to his mother and looks forward to the time he can be reunited with her, though he has some realization that she is not as dependable as his father. He definitely looks forward to seeing his father toward whom he is quite affectionate and from whom he receives a regular weekly allowance.

"We have included both parents in our planning for Clyde but have noted that Mrs. S. is so disturbed and confused that she cannot assume consistent responsibility for the boy and has not kept appointments with our worker regularly. However, she has been quite well satisfied with the care we have given him although she is still insistent upon taking him home as soon as her circumstances change. At present she is in the midst of divorce proceedings, undertaken at her expense and with Mr. S.'s consent, where she expects to receive the boy's custody. . . .

"Although we have found Mr. S. to be somewhat unstable, he has shown very regular interest in Clyde, not only visiting him regularly, but in providing him with spending money and clothing beyond our allotment. In our contact with Mr. S. he has indicated that this was made possible by Clyde's placement in neutral surroundings. Mr. S. is pleased with Clyde's progress and would like him to remain under our care for some time to come, rather than be reunited with Mrs. S. Yet he has not been ready to take any action in gaining custody of the boy for fear that this would not be granted because he is the guilty party in the divorce proceedings.

"It is our opinion that Clyde would benefit from continued removal from his parents since neither one is better able to care for him than at the time of his remand to us. We believe that we could help the boy to an even better personal adjustment and understanding of his familial situation if he remained under our care, although we know that this plan would probably be opposed by Mrs. S. If you should deem it to his welfare to follow out our recommendation, we would be willing to accept Clyde on commitment."

The court was happy to accede to the request for commitment in Clyde's interest. It means that he will remain at this excellent institution until he has made a satisfactory adjustment. If at that time neither parent is able to give him adequate care, Clyde will be ready for a foster home.

Here it is seen how adverse parental influence can cause personality distortions in a child. The case also demonstrates the need for flexible intake policies, just as there is need for flexibility in field practice among social agencies.

RONALD W.

His parents, older brother and sister indulge Ronald, 15, who truants and keeps failing in all his subjects. He dislikes school, where he is in 8A grade, and expresses a desire for employment. Occasionally he does odd jobs but spends most of his time with older truants in movies or loitering in candy stores and on street corners. Two years ago Ronald was in an accident, during which he received shrapnel wounds on his left foot and right hand. After a month's hospitalization he returned home as cured, but according to his mother, he has been "acting strange" ever since. He screams during the night and suffers from frequent and severe headaches. Both parents work, Mr. W. as a truck driver and Mrs. W. as superintendent of the large apartment building in which the family lives. The father believes Ronald is the mother's problem, and she in turn makes excuses for him when he absents himself from school.

When Ronald was referred to the court for excessive absences, the judge ordered full medical, psychological, and psychiatric examinations to aid him in deciding upon a course of action. Ronald was found to be well developed and well nourished, with height and weight above average, but poor posture. He scored an I.Q. of 95, average intelligence, solving fables at a 12-year level, failing with inductive reasoning at 14 but succeeding with factual and arithmetical reasoning at the 14-year level. His planning was inferior and his arithmetic achievement was equal to grade 5, showing considerable scholastic retardation. However, on the Stenquist assembly test he was equaled or exceeded by only 3.8 per cent of boys his age, indicating very superior mechanical ability.

In psychiatric interviews Ronald was cooperative and willing to discuss problems. He was tense and nervous, revealing some apprehension. One reason he dislikes school is that he is too old for his class. He was critical of his academic course and would like instead to be taking instruction in sheet metal work and electric wiring. He admitted to trouble at home and related this to his truancy. With his mother constantly worrying about money, she sometimes yells at him. Then he loses his temper and leaves home for a few days. He repeatedly apologized for his mother, wishing she did not get so excited. Ronald denied that he still has nightmares, contending these lasted only for a short while after his release from the hospital. He evinced great affection for Mr. W.

The psychiatrist concluded that Ronald is a rather unstable boy whose home does not offer him sufficient security. Probation was advised, with referral to an orthopedic clinic for advice concerning posture, referral to a mental hygiene clinic, since Ronald seems ready for help, and a complete change of school program to aid him in developing his mechanical ability. Admission to a recreational center would also be desirable. The court in cooperation with the educational authorities carried out these suggestions. Reports received at intervals during the two semesters which followed disclosed that Ronald is attending all his classes with regularity and is deriving special satisfaction from his instruction in sheet metal work. He is no longer a problem either at school or at home.

Prognosis for Ronald is favorable, since he received timely help which he was able to utilize satisfactorily.

CARL D.

Carl was almost 16 and in the first term of high school when he was brought into court as a chronic truant. While his school achievement was average in elementary school, his record card indicates emotional instability. He dislikes school and talked of entering a vocational high school. Carl's teachers and social workers who have known him feel his difficulties stem from a disturbed family life. Mr. D., devoted to his two children, is ineffectual in his efforts to guide them. After intermittent periods of desertion and return, Mrs. D. left the home permanently when Carl was 12 and his sister, Mildred, was 11. Mr. D. then divorced his wife. During these times he could not care for the children. He placed them in separate foster homes because from the time they were tiny there has been intense friction between the two children. Neither really accepted the foster home.

Since the divorce Carl and Mildred have lived with their father, who operates a small dry-cleaning store. Occasionally they visit their mother but, according to Mr. D., both are upset after these visits. In 1943 Carl ran away from his father. He soon returned and to keep him out of trouble Mr. D. keeps Carl at the store. This seems to make him restless and unhappy, so his father is at a loss to know what to do. Mr. D. has contemplated remarriage but hesitates, he says, because his new wife might not be acceptable to the children.

In response to a request from the judge, Carl was studied in the court clinic. He is fairly well nourished and developed, tall and thin, with above-average height, and in good physical condition.

On the psychometric tests Carl scored an I.Q. of 110. He was cooperative and interested in the procedures. The psychologist described Carl as a boy with generally superior intelligence, with particularly good powers of reasoning, auditory memory, and use of language. His weakness is in his capacity for abstract visual manipulation of nonlanguage material, in coping with spatial relations. His visual memory is not up to average, but when a problem with concrete objects is placed before him he handles it in superior fashion. In reading tests Carl demonstrated his highest level of achievement. Lack of practice has lowered his arithmetic score abnormally. He has capacity for completing a high school course in normal time, despite the fact that he has failed his four terms of high school. Poor visual memory and difficulty with abstract spatial relations may make advanced mathematics hard for him, but otherwise his ability is generally superior.

Carl was friendly in the psychiatric interviews. He made a good impression, but lacked force, was vague and concealed his feelings. When oportunities for psychiatric assistance were explained, he responded that he is confident he can manage himself. The diagnosis made was mild instability in a boy of superior intelligence. Probation was advised, with mental hygiene clinic treatment kept in reserve. The court abided by these recommendations. Carl returned to school and improvement was noted in his conduct and marks. This continued even after he was discharged from court supervision for excellent attendance and conduct. At the end of the school year Carl appeared voluntarily and asked the court for a letter of reference as to his character in order to obtain a farm job. A letter of recommendation was written, Carl secured the job, and having reached 16, he elected to remain with the farmer after the summer vacation period ended.

Prognosis for Carl is also favorable due to his superior intelligence and lack of any extreme emotional deviation, together with his capacity for adjustment in a changed environment which he himself arranged.

VERNA T.

Verna is 15 and in the third term of high school. She has an older sister who is a clerk and a younger brother who is in 7A.

Mr. and Mrs. T. are well thought of in the community; he is a probation officer, and she keeps busy in the home. When Verna began truanting her father took her to a guidance clinic for help. There Verna cried bitterly and told the interviewer that Mr. T. beat her unmercifully and never permitted her to have any friends. As Verna continued at the clinic she repeatedly mentioned that her father was inhumane to her and her mother, and she, Verna, was afraid to live at home. Meanwhile, her absences from school mounted until she was referred to the court as a truant.

Verna seemed very unhappy and related episodes which indicated the desirability of psychometric and psychological examinations for her, with informal observation of her parents. They were seen at the court clinic together and separately. Verna was found to have superior intelligence with symptoms of mild instability. Her accounts of her father were discovered to be fallacious. Mrs. T. was the really disturbed individual in the family. She suffered from feelings of deep anxiety and fear. Verna was inclined to blame her father for this and felt she was "getting back at him" by making false accusations against him. Verna identified strongly with her mother and did not like to be apart from her for long.

When psychiatric service was offered to Mrs. T. and Verna, they were unwilling to accept it. It is recognized that Verna's truancy is related to her mother's mental disturbance, but there is little that can be done in the circumstances. After a short interval the family moved from the state and the court had no alternative but to close its case.

Prognosis for Verna is poor despite her superior intelligence, since neither she nor her mother is willing to accept help and without help their difficulties will increase, not diminish.

LESLIE N.

Leslie, 15½ years of age, is the youngest of five children and the only one of school age in his family. Two older brothers are in military service, one sister is married and lives away from home; one employed brother and a sister live with Leslie and their mother, a widow. Leslie repeated 4B grade and is now spending his third term in 7A. For the past two years Leslie's absences have become increasingly noticeable, although his conduct has always been good, both in school and at home. On the school health card it is noted that Leslie does not appear well, has bad posture, is nervous, and had an operation for brain trouble nine years ago.

When Leslie was brought into court for truancy the judge ordered physical, psychometric, and psychiatric study of Leslie as a guide in deciding what to do in his behalf. Medical findings were negative except for underweight and numerous dental caries. A balanced diet and rest were prescribed. Leslie scored an I.Q. of 87, with a classification of dull normal to low average. A marked fluctuation in mental efficiency was apparent. He showed poor perception and poor social comprehension. There was a definite impairment in abstract learning ability. Scholastically, he read at fourth-grade level, spelled at second-grade, and was able to do arithmetic of the sixth grade. He displayed good manual dexterity.

On the psychiatric examination, Leslie was seen to be extremely immature, suggestible, unstable, impulsive, dependent, easily influenced—an essentially inadequate make-up with little insight. It is possible that the older, more stable brothers may give him some added help and encouragement to refrain from antisocial behavior. It was plain that Leslie would not benefit from further academic instruction, but he might adjust better in vocational courses. Although he possesses some manual dexterity, it is not sufficient for attaining his ambition of airplane mechanic. It was suggested that Leslie be encouraged to obtain an employment certificate at 16 and be directed into routine factory work.

Accordingly, the court arranged a school transfer for Leslie and facilitated the issuance of a work permit by making sure that necessary dental work was performed prior to his sixteenth birthday, and stressed the value of improved nutrition and regular hours.

It is likely that Leslie will drift from one unskilled job to another because of his instability, his inability to learn a skilled trade, his impulsiveness and his essentially inadequate make-up. Unless he begins to consort with criminals, the chances are that he will be law abiding, for his attitudes are not antisocial.

NICK F.

Nick, 13 years old and a pupil in 6A, lives with his mother and stepfather, who is now in the army. An only child, born out of wedlock, Nick has done quite as he pleased from the time he was a very small boy. Ever since his father deserted when Nick was 6, Mrs. F. has worked outside the home as a garment operator. The F.'s occupy a three-room apartment in a residential area that has ample facilities for recreation. Yet Nick has spent most of his time in the company of older boys roaming the streets and frequenting movies. He has always been well supplied with money by his mother who is overindulgent. In a mood of exasperation with him when he was 10, she filed a petition of delinquency against him, alleging that he was incorrigible and ungovernable. The judge made no finding but referred Nick to a guidance agency whose personnel was unable to reach him.

Due to Mrs. F.'s employment, Nick has been left mainly to his own devices. After she would leave for work he would take advantage of this lack of supervision and truant. On the rare occasions he attended school Nick annoyed other children and insisted upon always having his own way. If his teacher attempted to correct or admonish him, he became impudent and surly. On the school record card carious teeth and enlarged, swollen tonsils were marked.

After several periods of prolonged truancy, Nick was referred to the court. The judge then called upon the court clinic for advice, meanwhile remanding Nick to a temporary shelter for several weeks in an effort to bring him to a realization that his truancy was a serious matter. A report of his stay in the shelter contains significant items. He got along extremely well with the other boys there. At first he was shy and self-conscious, but later made friends and took part in programs of games and sports. However, in his contacts with the social worker he was like a different child—extremely tense, strained, and overanxious not to reveal too much. Anything pertaining to his home could not be discussed with him as he quickly became defensive and "touchy." His relationship with his mother seemed to be a constant source of considerable anxiety and insecurity for him and threw him into a turmoil. He clings to her, yet is aware of her shortcomings which he tries to deny since he cannot face these. He assumes that he has to shield and protect her, but is conflicted in his thinking about her.

Mrs. F. was seen to be a very upset and emotionally deprived person. She clings to Nick and pushes him into a possessive relationship which brings confusion and guilt. She demands an emotional satisfaction from him which she otherwise cannot obtain. She is conflicted and overanxious about "the mess" she has made of her life and has found herself in situations she no longer can bear. Desperately Mrs. F. wants to believe that Nick knows nothing of her life, his illegitimacy, her fears that her present husband will not want to return to her. It is quite unlikely that Nick is as unaware of these matters as she hopes, for his inability to talk about her except to defend her and his other behavior suggests conflict, not lack of awareness. Both Nick and his mother have a capacity to relate themselves to a case worker or a psychiatrist.

Physically, Nick is a precociously developed adolescent who has the appearance of a boy three years older than he is. He was seen to need glasses, dental care, and a tonsillectomy. On the psychological tests he obtained an I.Q. of 84, which is not fully representative as he scatters into the 14-year level in abstract and matter of fact reasoning, indicating that he is at his own age in terms of thinking but functioned poorly on the tests because of lack of interest and lack of application to concentrated thinking. His scholastic achievement is at 4B level, indicating marked educational retardation. On mechanical tests he scored below average. In the psychologist's opinion Nick possesses average intelligence but has been functioning below his best level of endowment because of emotional factors.

Nick impressed the psychiatrist as closely attached to his mother, a warm, well meaning boy whose maladjustment at school was due mainly to a lack of supervision and to a precocious physical development that made him wish to associate with older boys and caused him to resent being in classes with smaller boys. There was no evidence of any overt antisocial leanings and nothing vicious in his personality. The psychiatrist encouraged Nick by letting him know that he is by make-up suitable for a business career and that in line with this he should acquire greater facility in the three R's and a broader grounding in general school subjects before he reaches 16. An effort was made to implant insight into his responsibility to himself, to his mother, and the community in terms of school attendance and effort. He promised to exercise greater self-control and to desist from the infantile habit of employing his school money to gravitate into movies.

The clinic suggested that Nick be tried in an opportunity class of 8B with bigger boys and that when he reaches 15 he should be transferred to a vocational high school. A school adjustment was arranged by the court, including remedial instruction in reading and arithmetic, together with medical and dental care. Nick and his mother continued to attend the clinic for several months and derived help from their talks with the psychiatrist. Reports from the school show that Nick has been making considerable progress, and the court believes the prognosis for him is good.

Prognosis for Nick does appear favorable, as he was able to utilize psychiatric help and he has shown no evidence of antisocial tendencies.

TOM R.

Since he was 10 years old Tom, now 14 and a pupil in 6A grade, has been known to Children's Court. The first charges were truancy, running away from home, and riding busses all night in the company of an adult with a psychiatric record. Probation did not help Tom, who again was charged with excessive truancy. The family received public assistance for eleven years prior to Mr. R.'s enlistment in the Navy. He never remained on any job for long, often deserted his family, was a heavy drinker, and appeared to be thoroughly irresponsible and unreliable. At one time he was in the psychiatric ward of Bellevue Hospital for chronic alcoholism and a head injury. Mrs. R. had filed several petitions against him for drinking and desertion but never pressed these charges. Tom's younger brother had been ill from birth and died in a state school for mental defectives at the age of 7. Mrs. R. seemed dull and uncooperative.

Tom has been a behavior problem for years and a focus of conflict between his mother and father. Tom was in two serious automobile accidents; in one he sustained a broken leg and head injuries on being struck by an automobile after hitching on a streetcar. Last year he suffered a severe stomach injury and spent three months in a hospital. Mrs. R. told the court that since the last accident Tom has been highly nervous, is unable to control his bowel movements, and that when it happens in school he is ashamed to return and wanders away from home for days at a time. In all, he has run away from home nineteen times. Mrs. R. apparently identifies Tom with her husband. She repeatedly tells the boy that he is as bad as his father; this Tom resents. He emphasized to the court worker that his father was very good to him, often played with him, helped with his homework, and he misses his father a great deal.

To guide the court in assisting Tom, he was remanded to Bellevue Hospital Psychiatric Division for study. Medical findings were essentially negative, except for left undescended testicle. Neurological examination showed dilation of pupils with convergence. Skull x-ray was normal. Blood Wassermann was negative. The medical history included a head injury at eight, with several fractures and cerebral concussions. Psychometric tests indicated Tom is functioning on a deteriorating intellectual level. He received an I.Q. of 78 on the Bellevue intelligence test and was classified as of borderline intelligence. On the Monroe spelling test he graded at 1.9, and on the Stanford reading tests at 3.9.

No psychotic or neurotic traits were observed, but during his stay in the hospital he was seen to be hyperactive and restless. It was thought that this hyperkinesis may be related to his previous head trauma. With the unfavorable home situation and Tom's history of chronic truancy, it was the psychiatrist's opinion that he should not be returned home but instead should be placed in an institution for normal boys. This recommendation was followed by the court, and in reports from the institution Tom is making slow but steady progress.

Although some progress has been made by Tom, the prognosis for him is not very favorable because of his deteriorating intellectual functioning, which with his hyperkinesis may point to the development of an organic brain disorder, but at least in a good institution he has more of a chance for stable living at this time than he would have in his home.

EDWARD F.

Edward, 14 and in the 6A grade, was brought into court for habitual truancy. Throughout his school life he has truanted but persistently so for the last two years. On his health card there are notations of nervousness, undue restlessness, nail biting, speech defect, stammering, squinting, sinusitus, and frequent stomach-aches. When attending classes his deportment is excellent. He gets along well with other children, both in school and in the neighborhood. Four months previously his mother had died. She was described as a fine housekeeper and an affectionate mother who was overprotective of Edward, her only son. Since her death he has lived with his grandmother, his father, a longshoreman, and a married sister, Alice. Mary, Edward's other married sister, was once a patient in a state hospital for the mentally ill, with a diagnosis of dementia praecox, catatonic type. She was known as shy, sensitive, and seclusive. Edward is said to have a warm feeling toward his parents and his home.

The judge ordered that Edward be examined in the court's clinic to see what suggestions the psychiatrist might have for him. Medical findings were negative except for undernourishment. Edward obtained an I.Q. of 102 on the Terman tests. He reacted slowly, concentrated well, and displayed good reasoning ability. Scholastically he showed a severe reading disability, his reading comprehension being at the 4B level. During psychiatric interviews Edward was pleasant, friendly, spoke readily, and tried to create a good impression. He was tense, restless, and laid much stress upon his stammering, which he blamed for his truancy as he is ashamed to speak before the other children, especially when he is called upon to recite.

When the psychiatrist talked with Edward about his having to face his problems in a constructive manner, he agreed in an intelligent and appreciative way with suggestions given him. He stated that he has made up his mind to attend school regularly and now that he does not have to sit continuously in one room as his classes will change every hour, he expects to be better satisfied.

Probation was recommended, with a program of remedial instruction in reading and a full, well balanced diet. Edward therefore was placed on probation and arrangements were made with the school for remedial instruction. He has returned to school and there are no more complaints of truancy.

Prognosis here is regarded as favorable, since Edward has a capacity to use help, has normal intelligence which he can be encouraged to utilize, is comparatively well integrated, and his conduct is good.

The Markedly Unstable Child

GLADYS A.

Gladys, 14 years of age and in 8A grade, was brought into court for chronic truancy. She has two brothers, Mike, 16, and Leonard, 8, and a sister, Martha, 12. Their father died of tuberculosis five years ago after a long period of chronic alcoholism. On several occasions he was carried into psychiatric wards suffering from delirium tremens. Both Gladys and Leonard have been hospitalized for arrested tuberculosis and both have been behavior problems for a long time. Their mother, who scarcely understands English, cannot control them and has expressed a desire to have them placed. All of the children are disrespectful to her; their continual quarreling has kept the apartment in a turmoil. Gladys' late hours at dance halls and movies were a source of anxiety to Mrs. A. A private family agency sought to aid her but found her not desirous of help.

Gladys was remanded to a temporary shelter, and examinations were ordered to be performed in the court clinic. Medical findings were essentially negative, except for impaired vision and nervousness reflected in tremors of the fingers, general restlessness, and tension. Gladys scored an I.Q. of 85, indicating low average intelligence. However, she had been away from school so long that her rating could not be regarded as representative, especially as she was not functioning at her best ability. Her achievement on abstract reasoning approximated her age level.

Psychiatric interviews revealed Gladys to be markedly unstable, impulsive, and restless. She is incapable of determining her conduct intelligently and protecting her health. She has been associating with and has been dominated by older, undesirable companions with whom she visited dance halls until 3 to 6 A.M. She dislikes school, does not know the work, and makes half-hearted offers to return to school. But since she can not control or recognize her conduct sufficiently for her own best interests, she is not dependable and can not fulfill her promises or her momentary resolutions. She is not fundamentally antisocially minded or vicious but is inconsiderate and indolent. With a diagnosis of behavior disorder in a markedly unstable adolescent, the psychiatrist recommended that Gladys be committed to a protective institution. The prognosis seemed good on a long-time basis under a program of stabilization and rehabilitation. This recommendation the court followed, and reports received point out that Gladys is making a favorable adjustment within the institution.

With skilled supervision and training over a substantial period, Gladys can be helped toward a satisfactory life adjustment. Without these, her serious instability would lead her into constant trouble.

MARIE S.

Marie, 14, is in 7B grade. An only child born out of wedlock, she lived quite happily in a foster home from the time her father disappeared when she was 2 until her mother brought her to New York when she was 12. Here she made her home with her mother and her mother's present friend, Mr. O., who calls himself Marie's stepfather, although she detests him. Mrs. S. and Mr. O. both work in the same factory, leaving their apartment at 6 A.M. and returning at 6 P.M. Between these hours Marie has no supervision except on the rare occasions when she attends school. Mrs. S. regrets having removed Marie from her foster home and has tried to make her feel secure by indulging her desires for clothing, spending money, amusements, etc., but Marie has become more and more demanding and disobedient. Mrs. S. feels too attached to Mr. O. to give up her association with him, even though she realizes that Marie resents it.

Because of prolonged truancy, association with undesirable companions, and remaining out late at night, Marie was brought into court. There she was given several opportunities on probation, but when these proved unsuccessful, she was remanded to a temporary shelter while the court pondered her case. Just previous to her referral to court Marie had been examined in a child guidance clinic. There she was found to have an I.Q. of 106 on the Wechsler-Bellevue intelligence scale. She achieved a grade of 9.4 on the Stanford reading test, and a grade of 5.8 on the Woody-McCall arithmetic test. On the basis of her performance, the examiner was of the opinion that Marie's potential ability is somewhat above average, though she was functioning at a high-average level. He concluded that she was very much preoccupied with problems of adjustment outside school and that her difficulties in the classroom were a reflection of these. The clinic psychiatrist felt that placement was needed but not a foster home, as Marie was too conflicted for this. The court had tried to place Marie in a noncorrectional institution, but no such opening was available due to an absence of public facilities and intake restrictions and insufficient facilities among private organizations.

At the temporary shelter Marie made such an unsatisfactory adjustment that the director begged the judge to remove her at once. Extreme impulsiveness and hostility were reflected in her daily altercations and fights with the other girls. Staff members described her as acutely insecure and insatiably jealous. She could not bear to have another child receive adult attention or be in the limelight even momentarily; if this happened, Marie immediately provoked a fight with that child. If another youngster so much as brushed against her, Marie struck her. She cried, "It's no use. You can't do anything with me. My father and mother both had tempers like this." She insisted upon having her own way completely and seemed unable to bear any pressure to conform. When pressed, she would have a temper tantrum but when not upset appears to be a refined, well brought up child who is clean and neat. In periods of anger she uses foul language, is insulting and threatening. She gave an impression of being quite conflicted in her feelings for her mother. Her removal from her foster home probably hurt her far more than she can let herself realize.

Placement in a more controlled environment was recommended. Under the circumstances, the court had no alternative but to commit Marie to a correctional institution. No report has been received as to her adjustment there.

Prognosis for Marie is poor despite her normal intelligence, as her lack of a stable family life, her extreme impulsiveness and hostility hinder her adjustment. It is likely that she will be unwilling to use counseling help and will continue to fight efforts to aid her in or out of an institution.

Neurotic Patterns

Neurotic traits are found among a number of children who truant excessively. Although manifesting such habits as enuresis, undue fatigue, nail biting, temper tantrums, or nightmares, either singly or in various combinations, they have not developed specific neuroses which are deeper and more intense. Although their emotional disturbance is not so serious as that of neurotic children, nevertheless it is more serious than that of the unstable youth and, for preventive reasons, requires psychotherapy as promptly as possible. These reaction habits are usually traceable to faulty home conditions, sometimes complicated by learning disabilities. Scholastic retardation in turn aggravates the child's difficulties, so that unless therapy is accompanied by remedial instruction, his disturbance is heightened and psychiatric treatment alone is of little avail. When a child cannot develop good habits while remaining at home because destructive familial influences render him unaccessible to treatment, his placement is essential to prevent deterioration of personality. Case records include instances where children have retrogressed from instability through neurotic patterns to neuroses and finally to psychoses for lack of suitable home environment.

Whenever neurotic patterns are evidenced, medical, psychological, and psychiatric study is advisable for expert diagnosis and constructive planning. It may be done in an outpatient clinic if facilities permit. In particular cases a subsequent period of hospitalization may be necessary to rule out possible organic or psychotic factors. For the most part, outpatient clinical findings suffice. It is with the children having neurotic traits that much preventive work can be done as the prognoses for most of them are good, provided even a minimum of treatment is available. Many are intelligent and responsive and their emotional condition does not require prolonged care or institutionalization. As with other medical and psychiatric problems, the earlier a correct diagnosis is made and care obtained, the greater the opportunity for cure.

AGNES R.

After running away from home and obtaining employment as a waitress, Agnes, 15 and a pupil in 7B grade, was brought into court for prolonged truancy. She and a friend had been sharing a furnished room. The family, consisting of Mr. R., an elevator operator, Mrs. R., a nurse, John, 16 and a high school student, and Agnes, occupies a four-room apartment in an old tenement building within a congested neighborhood. There has been repeated conflict between the parents and the children. About three years previously Mr. and Mrs. R. were arrested for disorderly conduct during a quarrel. He is reported to abuse his wife and children and on several occasions threw them out of the apartment with the furniture. He and Mrs. R. often overindulge in alcohol. To the court worker Agnes revealed intense negative feelings toward her father.

To assist the court in helping Agnes, physical, psychometric and psychiatric study was ordered while she remained in a temporary shelter. Medical findings were negative. On the Stanford-Binet scale, Agnes scored an I.Q. of 86. She did not listen to questions and her replies were somewhat at random. A lack in reasoning ability was apparent, but she has a good rote memory for digits both reversed and direct at the superior adult level, which raises her I.Q. Her mental functioning is poor; for example, her arithmetic was at fifth-grade level.

Data obtained in psychiatric interviews proved helpful. Agnes was seen to be a nervous, tense child with occasional mannerisms. She talked volubly in a superficial way but expressed a definite feeling that her troubles were due mainly to her father, asserting that he permitted her no freedom to carry on a normal social life. When she fails to return home before 8 P.M. he becomes violent toward her, fights, breaks the furniture, and drinks. She is afraid of him and affirmed that her running away has been the only way she knew to escape from an intolerable condition. Agnes loves her mother and feels a marked degree of bitterness over her father's claim that she is not his child, as she thinks this reflects on her mother's conduct. Agnes recognizes her mother's rigidity concerning sex and found it hard to discuss sexual experiences. Finally Agnes mentioned that while she was away from home she went to a party, had too much to drink, and woke up the next morning in bed with a strange man. She also brought out that she has few friends, preferring to be by herself, has little ambition for the future but has some insight into her need for help and would like to continue at the clinic. A diagnosis was made of primary behavior problem, neurotic traits with a recommendation for clinic care.

The psychiatrist also saw Mrs. R., a dull woman appearing much older than her years. She shows the strain of overwork, together with the strain of emotional problems. While she does not openly reject Agnes, the 16 year old son is her favorite. At the same time that she stated Agnes is a "wonderful child," Mrs. R. also compared Agnes to Mr. R., stressing that Agnes looks and acts just the way Mr. R. does. It seemed possible that Mrs. R. has some guilt feelings about Agnes' conception, for the mother talked a great deal about the fact that when she was pregnant with the child Mr. R. kept insisting he was not the father, and, since that time, whenever he has temper tantrums he reproaches her with this. Her rigidity of attitude regarding sexual matters may be somewhat related to this; she announced that if Agnes had had sex relations when away from home, she, Mrs. R., would have Agnes placed in an institution. Later when it was explained to her that Agnes' sex experience had been accidental, Mrs. R. accepted it but insisted that no one but the judge and the clinic should know of this. Her feeling was one of shame and that it reflected on her as a good mother. At this point she seemed to have more insight into what the children had suffered because of their father's violence and said that the next time he had a temper tantrum she would establish a new home for them. In response to an inquiry she declared that Agnes had always been a sickly child, suffering from enuresis until she was 11.

Acting upon the advice of the psychiatrist, the court placed Agnes on probation and arranged for her and her mother to attend a mental hygiene clinic. At first some improvement was noted. However, when Agnes again ran away from home after Mr. R. had beaten her and his wife brutally, it was plain that the environment was precipitating Agnes' delinquent behavior and that she needed placement. It was felt that in a neutral environment she would be capable of a good adjustment. A place was found for her in a fine private institution with normal girls of her age group. Their reports show that Agnes is making steady progress and is happier than she has ever been.

It is likely that Agnes will adjust satisfactorily in the community after a period of time in this institution as she will obtain skilled help there and is not antisocial. She needs steady guidance and a relatively calm environment while developing new habits.

VINCENT C.

Vincent, 15 and a pupil in the 8A grade, has a sister, Gladys, two years younger; their parents had married when 16 and had been very unhappy together. Mr. C. has been irresponsible, remained away from home for several weeks at a time without explanation, gave up one job after another as being beneath him, and showed little interest in his children. Mrs. C., intelligent and alert, has had a number of extramarital relationships. After she gave birth to a child by a Mr. L., her husband left the home, later divorced her and remarried. She then had three other children whose paternity Mr. L. acknowledged. He and Mrs. C. talked of marrying, but since his return from army service he has been nervous and disinclined to be with her. Meanwhile, she is reported to have become exceedingly friendly with several other men. During these years Vincent and Gladys lived with other relatives and in orphanages. At one time her father sheltered Gladys but refused to have anything to do with Vincent on the ground that he always sided with his mother. For a while Mrs. C. was estranged from her mother and brothers, who disapproved of her conduct, but because Vincent was devoted to them she resumed her visits. Various social agencies had tried to aid her, but she refused their counsel and efforts.

Vincent, in trying to supplement the family income from public assistance funds, began to work after school hours and on holidays, turning all his earnings over to his mother. On each small task he was a steady and willing worker. As he became more aware of her irregular activities, he felt embarrassed about attending school and sought refuge in employment. When brought into court for habitual truancy, he said that his teachers questioned him about his home, particularly about Mr. L., and as Vincent did not like to talk about his family, he stayed away from school. At this time he and Gladys were living with their mother in a tiny, gloomy apartment, while their younger half siblings were in child caring institutions.

The court decided to have Vincent studied in a mental hygiene clinic and see what recommendations would be made for him. He was found to be in good physical condition and of average intelligence, with an I.Q. of 94 on the Bellevue scale, although retarded two years in arithmetic, due partially to his excessive absences. He demonstrated a high degree of dexterity and expressed considerable interest in obtaining vocational training. In psychiatric interviews he was unresponsive, but it was apparent that he was deeply concerned about his mother. Her instability and her mode of life kept him in a state of unhappiness and anxiety. Genuinely fond of her, he could not bear to accept her irregularities and fought against these. The resulting tensions were such that he could not keep his mind on school and feared inquiries about her.

Placement was recommended for Vincent in an institution for normal boys offering trade training and guidance. When it was discussed with him and his mother, neither objected; in fact, both welcomed the plan. Mrs. C. had noticed Vincent's attitude and seemed relieved that he would not be present to scrutinize or question her behavior, just as he was glad of a respite and a chance to start anew. The court thereupon effected a placement in which Vincent made a splendid adjustment. During a stay of a year and a half he learned to live a balanced life of study, work, and recreation, and became an electrician. Upon discharge he obtained skilled employment in his trade and found it enjoyable to maintain his mother, Gladys, and himself in a pleasant apartment.

Prognosis here appears good because of Vincent's steadiness, skill, strength of character and lack of any antisocial tendencies. Whatever his mother's conduct may be in the future, he is much more capable of coping with it. A number of persons connected with his case felt that the court should have penalized his mother. But with what results? Her dissolute habits were well developed, and she was not accessible to guidance or aid. Punitive measures would not have assisted either her or her children, for they would have been stigmatized by her arrest or imprisonment on a charge of contributing to the neglect or delinquency of her child. Even though it was recognized that her misconduct was the major causal factor in Vincent's truancy, retaliation would not help. However, to save him from being labeled a delinquent, a neglect petition was taken, for he was essentially a neglected child rather than a delinquent one.

MARIA S.

Maria, a pale, thin child of 14 enrolled in the 7A grade, has four older siblings who left home as soon as they reached an employable age to escape their mother's rigid domineering attitudes and actions. After years of marital friction, due mainly to her insistence upon spending family savings upon her imaginary illnesses, Mr. S. left the household and later disappeared, following a period of confusion and an attempt at suicide. Feeling a need to lie in bed most of the day, Mrs. S. depended upon Maria to prepare their meals and do the housework, so she formed the habit of remaining away from school and, because of her mother's insistence, did not mingle with other children, staying home practically all of the time.

When Mrs. S. and Maria were referred to the court because of the latter's school absences, the mother produced a doctor's certificate stating that Maria had been under his care for the previous three months receiving treatment for neurasthenia and suggesting that she be sent to a mental hygiene clinic for further treatment. Mrs. S. reiterated that she herself was very ill and needed a series of operations. Reports of her visits to clinics indicated that her complaints of gallstones, weak kidneys, and heart trouble were not borne out by medical examinations, and her requests for operations were not based upon medical opinion. She told the court that Maria knew enough already and did not need to continue at school; it was about time for her to be of some use in the house, especially as the older children had deprived the family of their earnings by leaving home.

In an effort to aid Maria, the court referred her to its clinic for study. She was found to be in good physical condition and graded low average in psychometric tests, with an I.Q. of 85. Scholastically she was retarded four semesters, attributable in part to her poor attendance record. During psychiatric interviews she was seen to be a quiet, meek, docile, and gentle child who was somewhat uneasy, apprehensive, and imbued with the idea that she was different from other children. She spoke of herself as being nervous, frequently ill, and having to urinate many times while at school or in the movies, adding that she would become dizzy whenever a teacher or children shouted. In the psychiatrist's opinion, Mrs. S. was keeping Maria in a dependent and dominated position, fostering inferiority and invalidism.

Immediate placement was recommended either with another relative or in a foster home. Despite Mrs. S.'s initial opposition to this plan, she changed her mind when it was pointed out that she could obtain a rest from responsibility for Maria's care. A married sister and her husband, both capable and deeply interested in Maria, offered her a home. The court accepted their offer on her behalf, awarding them custody. Steady improvement followed; Maria seemed to blossom out in her new freedom and security. There was no question about her school attendance, and her feelings of being ill, dizzy, and different from other girls soon disappeared in her new setting.

There is little possibility that Maria will be in further difficulty, for she is responding well to her new environment and has opportunities for wholesome development which she is ready and able to utilize.

EDMOND E.

Edmond was 13 and in the 7B grade when he was brought into court as a persistent truant. He is the eldest of three siblings whose parents entered into a forced marriage at the age of 17. The home was characterized by prolonged marital friction, complicated by discordant relationships with Mr. E.'s family until his death two years previously. Mrs. E. related to the court that her husband had been alcoholic, abusive, and irresponsible. She tends to see in Edmond's behavior the reflection of his father's family traits— his drunken paternal grandmother, his paternal aunt who was a delinquent, and his father's unstable youth and manhood. Edmond himself has expressed a desire to change his name so as to escape from the onus his father's name bears for him. For a long time he has been in conflict about his loyal and affectionate feelings for his father and his feeling that he must adopt his mother's attitude toward Mr. E. as a man who "deserved his death." At the same time that Mrs. E. tries to project the blame for Edmond's troubles on his father's family, she revealed feelings of rejection for Edmond and her other children, none of whom was wanted.

The family has been receiving public assistance since before Mr. E.'s death, as he rarely had been able to hold a job. Educational authorities described Edmond as defiant, sullen, inattentive, indifferent to his subjects, and resentful both of classroom supervision and of his mother's supervision. While truanting, he keeps away from his home, as his mother would then know of his school absences, roams the streets and seeks the company of other truants.

On referral to the mental hygiene clinic of a famous hospital for study, Edmond was found to be in excellent physical condition. On psychometric tests he scored an I.Q. of 87 in the Bellevue scale, with a wide range in the subtests. His functioning was uneven and he was under great tension trying to cope with problems beyond his emotional resources, so that his judgment suffered from constraint and lack of proper direction. Educational tests disclosed severe reading and arithmetic retardation, and this, together with his relatively low I.Q., indicates that his training should be along vocational lines rather than academic.

In psychiatric interviews Edmond was seen to be infantile in his behavior and attitudes. Although he talked freely when questioned, he rarely volunteered information spontaneously. Both his speech and his way of verbalizing were more immature than usual for his age group. During these discussions he occupied himself with drawing in a markedly compulsive way. He exhibited preoccupation with family problems and a sense of deep loss through the death of his father. It appeared obvious that his mother, though cooperative, has emotional difficulties of her own and has a mildly rejective attitude toward Edmond and the sister next to him in years. In spite of his feeling of rejection by his mother, he is deeply attached to her and is eager to help her financially. He is easily suggestible, but fundamentally he has a kindly disposition and with a little guidance should outgrow his present disturbance as his mild compulsive traits are susceptible to treatment. He expressed remorse and a willingness to admit his mistakes.

The psychiatrist recommended that Edmond should be encouraged to join recreational groups and receive mental hygiene aid in an institution having good activity programs. With Edmond's consent and that of his mother, the court placed him in an industrial farm school. He remained there approximately a year, achieving good subject and conduct grades. Then at his request he was discharged to his mother. Since then his school record has been satisfactory.

Prognosis for Edmond is good, since he received skilled help at a crucial period, and he has many fine traits which he will have more opportunity to exhibit after he leaves school. He will be more able to bear his mother's feelings toward him, and this will ease matters for him.

ALBERT A.

Albert, 10 and in the 5A grade, is the youngest of three brothers whose parents are rigid and strict in their attitudes. After Albert had been disorderly in school, attempting to strike his teachers and pouring ink on their clothing, he was suspended and referred to the court. His parents were hostile toward the educational authorities, accusing them of persecuting Albert because of his color. While they have been protective and defensive about the children outside the home, there they are severe and punitive. In the marital friction which has existed for many years, the children are made focal points of arguments and quarrels, with allusions to their never having been wanted. Mrs. A. is a good housekeeper who keeps the apartment clean and attractive. Mr. A. has been steadily employed in one place as a fireman for the past seventeen years and provides for the household to the maximum of his salary.

When Albert's conduct became very violent, the court remanded him to Bellevue Hospital Psychiatric Division for observation. Medical findings, including neurological, were negative. Albert was found to be well developed and well nourished, in good physical condition. On psychometric tests Albert scored an I.Q. of 93 and was classified as of low average intelligence, retarded in reading, spelling, and arithmetic. In psychiatric interviews he was anxious and depressed, finding it hard to talk about himself. He acknowledged it was difficult for him to keep up with the work of his class and then felt goaded into outbursts. He has trouble making friends and feels that people are not sufficiently sympathetic to him. In his view his teachers and his parents are too strict with him and expect too much of him, and it makes him uncomfortable. Albert is deeply attached to his home and expressed a feeling of warm affection for his family. On the ward he was well behaved and revealed no special problems except anxiety and defensiveness.

In the opinion of the examining psychiatrists, Albert's misbehavior was a neurotic reaction against too strict discipline and lack of sufficient affection in his home and against being overgraded and pushed too hard in school. They felt strongly that there is no basic reason why he should not get along well in his own home, in school, and in the community if his reasonable needs for affection, understanding, and proper grade placement were met.

Acting upon these findings and recommendations, the court, in cooperation with the Board of Education, arranged a transfer to another school for better classroom adjustment and counseled with his parents in his behalf. Six months later a report was received from the new school. His teacher commented, "Albert may have been a problem before he entered this school, but he has shown no signs of being one since." He is a leader in group instruction and feels that his group depends upon him for help. He responds eagerly to praise for his efficiency in handling the group and wants to retain his leadership. With considerable pleasure he has shown his A's in conduct and effort to his father, who has been making a real effort to be more companionable to his children. Albert, who now has a cheerful appearance and a hearty laugh in contrast to his former gloomy expression, told his social worker that he is happy and likes his life.

Prognosis for Albert is good, as fundamentally he is capable of a fine adjustment and now has opportunities which encourage rather than discourage him. He has received timely help.

MAURY R.

Maury was 13 when he was first known to the Children's Court as a neglected boy whose father, an alcoholic and a religious fanatic, was violently abusive to Maury, his three younger sisters, and Mrs. R. After an adjudication of neglect, Maury was placed in a private child-caring institution from which he ran away several times until that institution discharged him as a runaway. Upon his return to the city he worked as a dishwasher during late afternoons and evenings, gambled at night, and arrived home to sleep at 4 or 5 A.M. He would then sleep until noon and could not be induced to attend school. Because of this, Maury was referred to the School Part of Children's Court as a habitual truant. Immediately thereafter he ran away from home and refused to appear in court. A warrant was then issued; he was apprehended and remanded to a temporary shelter pending arrangements for psychiatric study, which, at that time could not be done within the shelter for lack of facilities. His behavior there was aggressive and disturbed, suggesting the advisability of a period of observation in a psychiatric ward for adolescents. Thereupon, when he was returned to court, arrangements were made for his admission to such a ward at an early date while in the interim he was remanded back to the shelter until a bed would become available in the hospital. During the second remand period Maury made concerted attempts to escape. He cried out that he was going crazy being in the building, expressed fear of being harmed by other boys in the group, and said he wanted to smash things and felt an almost uncontrollable impulse to choke a boy to death. He also expressed many fantasies about previous homosexual and heterosexual experiences. In view of these circumstances, the shelter authorities arranged for Maury's immediate admission to the adolescent ward of Bellevue Hospital Psychiatric Division on an emergency basis.

Medical findings, including neurological, were essentially negative. In psychometric study he rated high average to superior intelligence on performance tests, with exceptionally fine comprehension of spatial concepts. Verbal tests were not given him at this time, since he had had so many previous ones that it was felt he was too familiar with these. It was noted that he had scored a verbal I.Q. of 93 one year before in guidance clinic tests. Before that he had been placed in ungraded classes on the basis of examinations in which he had scored I.Q.'s of 79, 72, 71, 74, and 81. His verbal scores usually brought down his composite I.Q., with wide disparities between his verbal and performance ratings.

On psychiatric observation Maury was seen to be moody, sensitive, restless, stubborn, suspicious, and a follower. He made a good adjustment on the ward, kept out of trouble, and assumed a protective role toward smaller boys, but revealed an intense dislike of Negroes. The examining psychiatrists found Maury's neurotic reactions were due in a large measure to his feeling of insecurity. Since he responded well to praise and encouragement, they recommended probation with further psychotherapy in a mental hygiene clinic.

This recommendation the court followed, but it did not succeed. With no stability or encouragement for Maury in the home, he continued with his pattern of gambling, late hours, and school absences, adding thefts as he lost his earnings at poker. Nor could he be induced to keep any appointments at the clinic. Faced with these conditions, the court committed him to a state correctional institution when no private noncorrectional place would admit him.

The prognosis for Maury does not appear favorable, even though psychotherapy is available where he now lives. Whether such aid and a regular routine will help him sufficiently to overcome his destructive habits and implant constructive ones seems doubtful considering his associates there. Yet to allow him to continue as he had been going is no protection to him or society. It is very unfortunate that a public noncorrectional center was not available where he could have received intensive rehabilitation service.

ANTONIO C.

Antonio, almost 16, is the youngest child and the only boy in a family of four siblings, whose father is a varnisher earning $45 weekly, and whose mother takes pride in keeping their apartment clean and orderly. His parents and older sisters pamper Antonio, who was reported by school authorities to be sullen, sulky, and very stubborn. He bullied younger children and has been known to use coercive measures to take lunch money from them. He gambled in recreational rooms, spent the greater part of his time on the streets and in motion picture houses. If criticized, he became insolent and abusive. Antonio's school record card showed that he was retarded four semesters, repeating 1B, 7A, and spending his third term in the 8A grade when he was referred to the court as a habitual truant. It was learned that his eldest sister, now employed as a secretary, had been a patient in a state hospital for the mentally ill with a diagnosis of dementia praecox, catatonic type. After two years of treatment she was discharged as cured.

As a step in helping Antonio, the court ordered him examined in a mental hygiene clinic. Physically he was found to be in good condition except for many dental caries. On psychometric tests he achieved an I.Q. of 89, but this low average was not considered a true index of his innate intelligence. Although Antonio's general comprehension was borderline and his general information dull normal, the psychologist felt that the boy's innate intelligence was high average with functional retardation to a low-average level. He was lackadaisical, tended to evade exertion despite his wish to cooperate, and took the path of least resistance, giving up readily. When encouraged to further effort, he succeeded in tasks he had relinquished. There was considerable fluctuation in his mental efficiency. In abstract learning, in integration and rote memory, he rated as of high average intellect, but in social comprehension his score was low. Antonio told the psychologist that he would much rather work than attend school and expressed an interest in carpentry. Good manual dexterity was indicated.

The psychological findings were confirmed in psychiatric interviews. Antonio was found to be oversuggestible, careless, emotionally immature for his age, with marked feelings of inadequacy and flat affect. A diagnosis was made for him of average intelligence with functional retardation and conduct disorder, with neurotic traits such as nail biting, dependency, and tantrums. It was concluded that he would not benefit from further academic training; rather, he should be transferred to a vocational course emphasizing carpentry.

The court accepted this recommendation, arranged a school transfer in cooperation with educational officials and placed Antonio on probation. When he achieved excellent marks in both conduct and subjects, he was discharged from probation.

Prognosis here is good. It is not likely that Antonio will become involved in serious delinquencies, as his neurotic patterns are mild and he will receive sufficient satisfaction from gaining and using a skill to enable him to be law abiding. Then, too, as he reaches adulthood and becomes employed there will be less inclination on the part of his family to pamper him.

GEORGE L.

George, 16 and a pupil in the first term of high school, was the second youngest of six siblings whose father is a fireman and whose mother is an excellent housekeeper. Upon his referral to the court for excessive truancy, Mrs. L. reported that he had "infantile paralysis of the brain" when a small child and he sometimes told her that "everything goes black" before him. He was fearful, restless, nervous, with frequent nocturnal emissions. Five years previously he was struck in the head with a baseball bat and remained in the hospital four days. He refused to attend school, and although of an age entitling him to a work permit, he expressed no inclination to apply for one as he had no desire to work. He has been stealing money from his mother and on two occasions ran away from home. Although he has shown an I.Q. of 105 in group tests, he was retarded three terms and detested school.

George has suffered from uneven supervision and lack of parental control. His father, a reserved person, was harsh and unsympathetic toward George whereas his mother, dominating and aggressive, has been protective toward him. Because of religious differences and a clash of personalities, there has been considerable marital friction. Mrs. L. has felt bitter as a result of her own unhappy childhood when her stepmother rejected her and placed her away from home for three years. Mr. and Mrs. L. were anxious for George to complete high school, but they could not induce him to attend. Their home is neat, well furnished, and in a good residential area, with plenty of play space. There has been no difficulty with his elder siblings nor with his younger sister.

Because of his history of head injury and other factors, the court remanded George to Bellevue Hospital Psychiatric Division for observation. Medical examinations, including neurological, were negative except that the electro-encephalogram was somewhat unstable, but it did not reveal anything to indicate a convulsive disorder. In psychometric tests George achieved an I.Q. of 109 on the Bellevue intelligence scale, but his verbal score was much lower than his performance score, the former being 97 and the latter 118. His rote memory and ability to form new associations were impaired markedly; this was a type of defect which would interfere greatly with school work. Scholastically he was retarded greatly, reading at a fifth-grade level and doing arithmetic at a sixth-grade level. Under these circumstances his distaste for school was easily understandable. But why this retardation in a boy of normal intelligence?

On the ward George presented no problem in adjustment. Friendly and cooperative in interviews, he spoke freely of his truancy, claiming that he could not develop any interest in his school work, feeling restless and fidgety. While this might be due to his educational retardation, the question arose as to whether his restlessness and inability to concentrate might not be due to his head injury, but the neurological findings were insufficient to hold this factor responsible for his maladjustment. His scholastic retardation and difficulties in his thinking processes made ordinary academic school adjustment a problem. On the other hand, he was shown to possess definite manipulative ability. The examining psychiatrists concluded that George's main trouble was neurotic conflicts, especially in the sexual sphere. They recommended that he be encouraged to go to work but that if the court desired him to attend school a program of mechanical courses should be stressed.

In court discussions with George and his parents he expressed a desire to take a job as a mechanic's helper in a garage and learn to be an expert mechanic. This was approved and he obtained an employment certificate. Since he did well on his job and attended continuation school four hours a week, the case was closed and he was discharged to his parents.

George probably will make a good work adjustment, as he has a chance to use his mechanical ability. One wonders whether or not his head injury may have a later adverse effect. It would be well if he could receive complete neurological study at intervals.

ARCHIE M.

Archie, 13 and in the 7B grade, is the youngest of three siblings whose mother is a widow. The eldest daughter, a stenographer, and her husband, a bricklayer, share the M. home and support the family. Mr. M., who deserted his family four years before his death from alcohol poisoning, had had intermittent employment as a mechanic. Their relationships were quarrelsome and tense. Archie was described by his teachers as a quiet, furtive boy who felt that he could do as he pleased without fear of punishment for his misdeeds. On several occasions he purloined belongings of classmates; about three years ago he took money and a watch from a neighbor's house where he had gone to visit. By making restitution, the mother had prevailed upon the woman not to press charges. When truanting from school, he spent most of his time roaming the streets picking up junk which he sold for pocket money. From time to time he attached himself to a gang of older boys who made a practice of stealing to obtain money for gambling and treats. About once a week Archie would remain away from home, usually lounging about the tenement house in which his family lived and subsisting on milk and buns stolen from neighbors. One of them complained recently that he had stolen money from her again.

In school Archie has progressed regularly from grade to grade, although his conduct marks have been poor since his initial enrollment. Group tests gave him an I.Q. of 100. Although his scholastic retardation was not serious, he was not up to grade in either arithmetic or reading but had been indifferent toward remedial instruction. On his record card were noted a speech defect, general restlessness, and occasional earaches. After his truancy became excessive he was referred to the court.

When asked about Archie, Mrs. M. told the court that she believed there was something wrong with his brain as a result of repeated mastoidectomies, causing total deafness in one ear and cerebral pressure. No objection was offered to a remand for medical and psychiatric observation of Archie.

At the hospital medical examination, including neurological procedures, disclosed that in addition to having a very small head, Archie had operative mastoid scars with few antral cells present. An electro-encephalogram ruled out any brain pathology. On the Bellevue intelligence scale he attained an I.Q. of 90—low average—but this was not considered truly representative of his innate ability because of educational retardation—he was able to do only third-grade arithmetic and reading and fourth-grade spelling. On the ward he made a very satisfactory adjustment but revealed neurotic traits such as stammering, bed wetting, and nail biting, but he showed no evidence of delusions, hallucinations, or other psychotic symptoms.

The examining psychiatrists concluded that Archie's chief problem was marked scholastic retardation, making it impossible for him to do the work of his grade. They recommended that he be given a chance on probation with a special program of intensive remedial instruction. The court followed their recommendation and, in cooperation with educational authorities, arranged for remedial work in arithmetic and reading. There was a frank discussion with Archie and his mother regarding the necessity and value of benefiting from expert instruction. Subsequent reports from the principal showed that Archie has been responding well and at the end of the school year he was almost ready for a regular grade placement.

Prognosis for Archie is rather poor, since he lacks adequate supervision and his irregular activities are of long standing. It is unfortunate that psychiatric counseling service was not available for him.

RICHARD N.

Richard, 13 and a pupil in the 8A grade, was referred to the court after being suspended from school for repeated truancies, disobedience, and misconduct in class. Teachers were annoyed at his running out of the room when classes were in session, his use of vile language, talking aloud and whistling when others were reciting. Mr. N. had died two years previously of heart disease. For many years he had worked intermittently as a laborer, but had never been able to earn enough to support his family of sixteen, six of whom remained in the home. Public welfare authorities had granted supplementary relief for ten years and full relief since Mr. N.'s decease. Both parents had been considered dull and inadequate. Mrs. N. was very nervous and irritable as a result of menopausal changes and was unable to cope with her children. In agency contacts she was overprotective of them and overly dependent.

The court remanded Richard to Bellevue Hospital Psychiatric Division for full study before deciding his case. Medical findings, including neurological, were negative, as he was in good physical condition. In psychometric tests he achieved a high normal intelligence rating with an I.Q. of 110 on the Bellevue scale. Yet he was retarded three years in reading and one year in arithmetic, which would make his present grade placement difficult for him. He exhibited excellent manipulative ability, far above most boys of his age group.

On the ward Richard was at first overactive, noisy, quarrelsome, associating with the ringleaders in causing disturbances. Later his behavior improved substantially; he was cooperative and helpful, obviously trying to earn a good report. During psychiatric interviews he was responsive and coherent, explaining his truancies by stating that he had "gotten in" with other boys who remained away from school and he had formed a habit of being with them and doing whatever they did. Admitting that he has been a problem in class sessions, he expressed some remorse for this and hoped to do better. His constant attention-getting mechanisms were operable to the point of being annoying, and the psychiatrists believed that these accounted in large measure for his difficulties in school. Neurotic traits were observed, including overattachment to his mother, enuresis, nail biting, nightmares, and temper tantrums, but he had no psychotic symptoms.

Bellevue recommended that Richard be placed on probation, that he receive intensive psychotherapy in a mental hygiene clinic, and that he be given remedial instruction in reading and arithmetic. These suggestions the court accepted and arrangements were made, in cooperation with school authorities, for special instruction and referral to a psychiatric clinic. Richard attended regularly and some improvement was noted at school and in the clinic despite several relapses into his old habit patterns.

Prognosis for Richard is fair. It remains to be seen whether or not psychiatric counseling service can overcome the negative home influences to which Richard is subjected constantly.

BRYAN C.

Bryan, almost 16, was a student in the first term of high school and had two older siblings and a much younger stepbrother born of his mother's second marriage following Mr. C.'s death when Bryan was 2. His stepfather, Mr. T., has never assumed responsibility for him and has resented his presence in the home. As soon as the older siblings reached working age, they left the household and preferred to remain away. Ever since his initial enrollment in school Bryan has been a problem because of truancy, insubordination, and disruptive conduct in classes. Twice he was suspended for the latter offense. Associating with undesirable companions, he loitered on the streets and in subways. Upon his referral to the court for excessive truancy, it was noted that Bryan had a number of neurotic habits, including thumb sucking, shoulder tics, eye blinking, hand tremors, nail biting, and a speech defect.

The court learned that Bryan had had medical, psychological, and psychiatric studies in a fine guidance unit operated by a private agency. There he was found to be in good physical condition, of low average intelligence, with an I.Q. of 90 on the Bellevue scale, emotionally immature with neurotic traits, and in need of placement within a controlled environment. They had suggested a placement plan to his mother several years previously, but she had been uncooperative, very protective, and resistive to treatment for him, emphasizing that he was misguided and nervous but not delinquent and showing no real insight into his problems. Bryan was insecure socially, always doing things for his friends for fear of losing them and attempting to purchase friendship by gifts, yet feeling dissatisfied with the few friends he had. He revealed undue dependence upon his mother and was aggrieved at her again becoming pregnant as he did not relish having another stepsibling.

It was ascertained that the guidance clinic had continued its efforts to help Bryan, but their psychiatrist, who had confirmed the earlier findings, was convinced that Bryan could not utilize treatment until he was removed from the home and placed in a setting more favorable to his development. They offered to admit him to one of their institutions for normal boys where he would receive psychotherapy and take part in a rehabilitative program of education, recreation, trade training, and regularized living.

The court accepted their offer and Bryan was committed to their care. About six months later he wrote to the court that he liked being there and felt as though he were learning to live a new life. Official reports confirmed that his adjustment was satisfactory, and he was showing marked improvement.

It is likely that Bryan will be able to make a good adjustment after he leaves the institution, as he will be equipped with habits of regular living and a considerable degree of self-knowledge together with a skilled trade.

ANTHONY F.

Anthony, 15 and enrolled in an ungraded class, is the middle sibling with three older brothers and three younger sisters whose parents are hardworking, respectable, and strict. Their oldest boy had been an inmate of a state school for mental defectives, but they grieved for him and effected his release to them against the advice of its officials. Throughout his school career Anthony has received a uniform rating of D in all his subjects except shop. His truancies were many, since he spent most of his time attending movies or roaming the streets in company with other truants. When he was referred to the court for habitual truancy, an accompanying report noted that whenever he was in class he was nervous and unduly restless. His health card mentioned impaired vision, enlarged, diseased tonsils, and nail biting.

In an effort to help Anthony, the court referred him to a guidance unit of the Board of Education for study before making a decision in his case. There he was found to have above-average height and weight, poor posture, obstructed nasal breathing, indistinct speech, impaired vision, enlarged diseased tonsils, deviated septum, four badly diseased molars. His parents were informed of his need for medical care and letters of referral to clinics were given to Mrs. F. Both she and Anthony promised to cooperate in plans for medical treatment. In psychometric tests Anthony achieved a dull normal I.Q. of 90, with a higher score on performance tests than on verbal ones. Scholastically he was very retarded, as he could not read, recognized only part of the alphabet, and his arithmetic was at the second-grade level. Quite probably this partially accounted for his poor school adjustment.

But why was he so retarded educationally? The examining psychiatrist attributed these disabilities partially to neurotic traits which Anthony had developed in response to parental strictness, and partly to his physical defects, which have long needed correction. Lack of glasses alone has been a serious handicap to Anthony.

The guidance unit recommended strongly that medical care be obtained immediately, that Anthony be regraded and receive special remedial instruction by one of their psychologists. These suggestions were accepted by the court, which placed him on probation, saw that he and his mother followed out medical plans and encouraged him to attend the clinic regularly. Improvement followed, and at the end of the semester probation was no longer needed.

Prognosis for Anthony is favorable, since he is receiving the help he needs and he is utilizing it satisfactorily. In addition, he has shown no antisocial tendencies.

KENNETH R.

Kenneth, 12 and enrolled in the 5A grade, was referred to the court for excessive truancy. He is the youngest of six children, all of whom, except Kenneth, are adults. When he was brought in accompanied by his mother, his brothers and sisters were living in other states and because of family quarrels had no communication with Mrs. R., who had divorced their father ten years previously. He had remarried and seemed content to disassociate himself from his children. Periodically Mrs. R. would become embroiled with school authorities, seeking to have Kenneth transferred from one school to another for fancied slights. To public assistance visitors from the welfare department which maintained Mrs. R. and Kenneth she was hostile and abusive.

At the first court hearing she was so incoherent, obscene, and irrelevant that it was plain that she was suffering from mental illness. Hallucinations and delusions of persecution were expressed graphically and in detail. She was remanded therefore to Bellevue Hospital Psychiatric Division for observation and possible commitment to a state institution; Kenneth was remanded to a shelter pending study in the court clinic regarding his placement needs. At Bellevue Mrs. R. was found to be psychotic with a diagnosis of schizophrenia and, after a hearing in Supreme Court, was committed to a state institution for the mentally ill.

In the court clinic Kenneth was found to be underweight and undersized, with many carious teeth and in need of eyeglasses. In psychological tests he achieved an I.Q. of 76, which was not considered truly representative of his innate ability because of blocking and scholastic retardation. He cooperated but was tense and fearful. On the Stenquist scale he displayed excellent mechanical ability, being equaled or exceeded by only 11 per cent of boys in his age group. His retardation in school skills was serious, since he read at the second-grade level and did arithmetic at the fourth-grade level. During psychiatric interviews Kenneth appeared dull, repressed, and unhappy, the result of exposure to a very destructive environment throughout his life. Although he talked timidly about his activities, he blocked excessively on the subject of his mother, whose mental derangement has caused him to lead a nomadic, disturbed existence. When asked about his identical twin brother, Robert, who had drowned four years ago, Kenneth displayed feelings of regret and loneliness at the loss, but had a profound need of protesting that he had not been with Robert at the time of the accidental drowning, in the manner of one who had been held responsible. He told how they had fought together but made up in a minute, always played together and could not be told apart, except that he had a little mole on his hand.

Only when talking of his married sister, Helen G., did Kenneth smile or relax. He lived in her home during the previous summer and his memory of it was that of a place where the family was happy and enjoyed many pleasant activities. The only school subject he liked was shop in which he excelled. His mother had caused him to change schools so often that he never felt that he belonged in any. Recognizing his own physical weakness, he was somewhat asocial in his relationship with boys. A diagnosis was made of a neglected child having mild neurotic trends. It was recommended that if it were at all feasible, he should be placed with Helen and that his school program should be arranged so as to give him a maximum amount of trade training. The clinic offered to accept Kenneth for psychotherapy in an effort to help him overcome the results of his severe traumatic experience in his home.

At this point Helen appeared before the court, stating that while in a southern state living near her husband, who was in the army, she had received a letter from her mother imploring her to take Kenneth and release Mrs. R. from the hospital. Helen, a young, attractive woman who worked part time as a skilled operator and maintained a comfortable home for her own child of 3, begged that Kenneth be permitted to live with her. She was disinclined to accept her mother's illness, preferring to feel that it was only fatigue and a "rundown condition." Helen disclosed that of all the children she was the only one who was interested in their mother and willing to have anything to do with her.

As the court found Helen to be stable and deeply interested in Kenneth and that her home was adequate, he was placed in her care. Arrangements were made for a special school program and for his attendance at a mental hygiene clinic. Improvement followed until Helen obtained her mother's release, against the advice of the court. Since her condition was not susceptible of much improvement even while under treatment, Mrs. R. proved to be as destructive in Helen's home as in her own. Her obscenity and other revolting behavior kept the household in such turmoil that Mr. G. who, in the meantime, had been discharged from the army and had joined them, dispaired and left Helen. Driven by feelings of guilt and fear, she could not bring herself to the point of having Mrs. R. leave. When the court pointed out to Helen that she was endangering the welfare of her own child as well as of Kenneth and herself by continuing to harbor her mother, Helen finally realized that the best course was to return Mrs. R. to the hospital. By that time Helen felt that she could no longer be responsible for Kenneth, since her first obligation was to her own child and her husband, so she asked to be relieved of Kenneth. The court agreed with her and placed him in an institution with normal boys where he lives in a stable routine and is again showing some improvement.

Kenneth has been subjected to so many traumatizing experiences throughout his most formative years that it will be a miracle if he develops normally even though he has now been placed. His placement should have been made long ago.

NEIL M.

Neil, 15 and a pupil in the 8B grade, has been known to various branches of the court for the past three years because of habitual truancy. He is the second of three brothers whose father deserted the home after he had stabbed his wife for alleged infidelities. Although he does not visit them, he has continued to support his sons by working as a barber. Mrs. M., impatient and neglectful, seemed resentful of the boys' presence in the house, which she kept in a disorderly condition. Neil had attended a probationary school for a period with no resulting improvement in his truancy or his conduct, which continued to be graded D. During his absences he wandered about the streets, occasionally helping his mother with household tasks. On his health card there was a notation of a cardiac condition not warranting placement in a health class.

At his first court appearances Neil had been remanded to a psychiatric hospital for observation. There he had been found to be in good physical condition except for a slight cardiac murmur which did not preclude normal activity. In psychometric examination he achieved an I.Q. of 119 on the Bellevue scale, with a verbal score of 101 and a performance score of 131, classifying him as of at least bright normal intelligence. A sampling of his oral reading suggested a reading disability, and it was the psychologist's opinion that Neil had a special difficulty in symbolic learning and was four years retarded in scholastic subjects.

Psychiatric observations revealed Neil to be timid, self-conscious, very sensitive about his failures, with deep feelings of inferiority because of his reading disability. He feared making mistakes in class, felt other pupils were laughing at his poor scholastic achievement, so escaped by remaining away from school, thus further impairing his skills and creating a vicious circle. It was recommended that he receive special tutoring in reading and arithmetic and as much encouragement as possible to attend a psychiatric clinic for treatment concomitantly with the tutoring. Still he continued to truant and failed to keep clinic appointments.

Again Neil was hospitalized for observation in an effort to help him. Medical and psychometric findings were similar to previous ones, except for a slight deterioration in the I.Q., which still indicated superior intelligence. On the ward and in psychiatric interviews he was withdrawn, inactive, timid, and gave an impression of being much duller than he is, probably due to emotional blocking. No psychotic trends were elicited, but a few neurotic traits were manifested, such as nightmares and undue fatigue. At first uncooperative, he responded to psychotherapy, became more pleasant, smiled, seemed happier and entered into games, although he continued to express a great deal of anxiety and insecurity, which were attributed to his poor relationship with his parents and siblings.

The examining psychiatrists concluded that Neil's troubles were due chiefly to severe educational retardation, feelings of inadequacy, immaturity and lack of proper supervision and understanding in his home. They felt that he was neglected rather than delinquent because of the unsatisfactory home situation and his mother's lack of cooperation in not bringing him to the mental hygiene clinic for treatment. Again a special program of remedial instruction was advised, together with psychiatric follow-up for his neurotic traits, but this time placement was suggested instead of probation.

When placement was discussed with Neil and his mother, they protested strenuously and promised that the hospital's advice concerning school and clinic attendance would be followed. For the first time Neil showed a realization that it was folly for him to continue with his old patterns when he had intelligence enough to really do well at school, graduate from elementary classes at the end of the term, and then enter a vocational high school of his choice. The court acceded to his plea and gave him another chance on probation. This time it worked. He felt himself old enough to supervise his own attendance at school and his clinic appointments. He gained a degree of facility in reading under special instruction, proved responsive to psychotherapy and entered a high school giving courses in aviation trades. There he did well and was discharged from probation.

Neil probably will continue to make a good adjustment as he is receptive to psychotherapy and benefits from it. He has sufficient intelligence and maturity to change his patterns despite adverse home conditions and enjoys studies along the lines of his special aptitudes.

ANTONIO C.

Antonio, 15 and enrolled in the second term of an academic high school, is an only son with four older sisters who live with their parents, a well-to-do, uneducated middle-aged couple who arrived in this country twenty years ago. All of his sisters, together with their parents, have hoped that Antonio would become a professional man and have urged him to complete school as fast as possible, giving him a high allowance and frequent money gifts to spur him on toward their goal. Whenever he pleaded to be allowed to stop school and find a job connected with machines, they dissuaded him—his father by offers of an increased allowance, his mother by tears and resulting headaches, and his sisters by lavish gifts. After sporadic truanting and failures in his subjects, Antonio began remaining away from school for weeks at a time, drifting into moving picture houses, pool halls and candy stores. When in classes, he was well behaved and alert.

Upon referral to court for habitual truancy, Antonio was studied in a guidance unit. Medical findings were negative, and on psychometric tests he was classified as of average intelligence with an I.Q. of 101 and an unusually high degree of mechanical aptitude. During psychiatric observation he manifested certain neurotic traits, including feelings of inadequacy and inferiority, undue fatigue, and slight depression. He was pleasant, cooperative, and displayed initiative and dependability. It was concluded that he was reacting against family pressures, and needed encouragement in developing his manipulative ability. This was discussed with his parents and sisters, who reluctantly relinquished their dreams for his academic training and consented to his desire for a transfer to a vocational high school, feeling that unless they did he might become involved in serious delinquency. Improvement followed almost immediately upon his transfer to a program of instruction in mechanics and a lessening of family tension regarding his future career.

Antonio became delinquent because of family pressures; as soon as these were eased his conduct improved markedly. Prognosis for Antonio is very good, since it was possible to remove the primary causal factor producing his misconduct. To try to impose family aspirations upon a child in direct contradiction to his own abilities breeds trouble and disappointment.

Chapter IV

NEUROTICS AND PSYCHONEUROTICS

THE CASES presented in this chapter represent children who are suffering from severe emotional disturbances, including feelings of anxiety and depression, some with schizoid features, and those whose mental deviation is more pronounced than a neurosis and is termed a psychoneurosis.[1] The latter can be said to border on the mentally ill. Usually their home life and school life are thoroughly unsatisfying to them and their families are characterized by irregular behavior patterns. Most of them require intensive psychotherapy and can benefit substantially from it. At times treatment in an outpatient center while they are residing at home suffices, but in other instances adverse familial circumstances impede recovery and necessitate placement.

CLARK M.

Clark, 15 and a pupil in the fourth term of a vocational high school, is the younger of two brothers. Their father, an alcoholic, committed suicide twelve years ago. Their mother, a telephone operator, was nervous and fidgety. After absenting himself from school for an entire semester and most of the previous one, Clark was referred to the court for habitual truancy. He had a fair record in elementary school and a commendable one the first-year

[1] See Lawson G. Lowry, *Psychiatry for Social Workers*. New York, Columbia University Press, 1946. O. S. English and G. H. J. Pearson, *Common Neuroses of Children and Adults*. New York, W. W. Norton & Co., 1937.

terms of high school. Lately he expressed pro-Nazi opinions, shocking his classmates by the intensity of his remarks. On his health card were notations of bronchitis, underdevelopment of sex organs, and possible glandular dysfunction. Mrs. M. told the court that when Clark became excited he would run a temperature and "cough up lumps of blood."

When Clark refused to attend an outpatient clinic for examination and possible treatment, he was remanded to Bellevue Hospital Psychiatric Division. Physical study showed that Clark was tall and well developed, except that he had rather small genital organs for his size and age. Examination of the sella turcica, which occasionally reveals pathology explaining such deviations in the growth of the genitals, was negative. Thorough tests of his lungs revealed no positive findings, except that x-ray of the chest showed evidence of healed lesions in one lung. In psychometric tests Clark achieved a composite I.Q. of 86 on the Bellevue scale, with a verbal score of 96, and a performance score of 79, classifying in the dull normal intelligence group.

On the ward Clark was friendly and cooperative. In psychiatric interviews he was quite open and friendly; he admitted his truancy because he did not like his school, adding that he was now ready to return, as he realized that he should finish high school. In the opinion of the examining psychiatrists Clark was a neurotic child who felt exceedingly insecure, fearful, inferior to others, and sensitive about his small genitalia which probably accounted for his fear and anxiety. His belligerent expressions were considered to be a reaction to his feelings of inadequacy. They believed he would be able to adjust satisfactorily in the community and, therefore, recommended that he be placed on probation.

Their advice was accepted by the court, which also arranged for his referral to a mental hygiene clinic. Clark returned to school, attended the clinic for a six months' period, during which he received reassurance as to his organs and developed insight into his problems. It is expected that he will graduate with his class.

It is likely that Clark will make a good adjustment, since he is receiving the help he needs.

SAM A.

Sam, 15 and in the 8B grade, is the eldest of three siblings whose father is a skilled garment worker and whose mother remains at home. David, the younger son, has been hospitalized since a serious attack of infantile paralysis almost two years ago, and his condition has been a considerable emotional strain to Mrs. A. When Sam was referred to the court for habitual truancy, he and his mother were interviewed separately. She spoke of her deprived childhood and that of her husband. She had to start working at 14, and he at 10. She had hoped to become an actress and still believed that she would have made a very successful one. She had felt like "killing" Sam many times when he was a baby as he had been cranky and tearful, and afterwards she had not wanted any more children. Following David's birth she had had a "nervous breakdown."

Sam was obese as a child and has been receiving injections which his mother felt were worthless, although he lost seventeen pounds as a result of these. He spoke of frequent undefined fears of his health, of his hatred of baths, fondness for old clothes, dependence upon cigarettes and cigars, and his fondness for two older boys. He admitted that he had been arrested along with them after stealing typewriters. No court action had been taken against them as the owner declined to prosecute in view of their youth. When he was younger Sam stole from 5 and 10-cent stores, "just for the thrill," but after he was caught three or four times he had become frightened and ceased. Just after his brother became ill Sam had become quite violent at home, breaking furniture and windows. Following a brief period at a hospital he had been allowed to return home.

On several occasions he has tried to run away to Florida but was returned home by the police. He revealed feelings of guilt toward his father, who was serious-minded, with old-world ideas, and who felt that beatings would help Sam. Frequently he mentioned his intense hatred of policemen and his dreams of killing them and seeing his parents and siblings dead. Once when he was about 6 he discovered his parents having sex relations; this "bothered" him for years. He hated his mother's nagging and has identified some of his troubles with her so that when teachers scolded him he walked out of the classrooms.

After weighing the pros and cons, the court remanded Sam to

Bellevue Hospital Psychiatric Division for a period of observation. He was found to be well developed and well nourished, having no physical defects. Neurological findings were negative. In psychometric tests Sam rated as of average intelligence with an I.Q. of 105 on the Bellevue scale. His Rorschach pattern suggested carelessness, lack of effort, easy, illogical rationalizations, and a great amount of fear confined mainly to the sexual sphere. On the ward he was easy-going, neglectful, and engaged in many mischievous activities. Fraternizing with many patients, he was sociable and friendly but not helpful. In psychiatric interviews he showed a very fluctuating type of behavior. At times he was cooperative and seemed to tell the truth; other times he was sulky, resistive, and hostile. When asked about the reasons for his truancy, he was very evasive.

Sam gave a history of an intact home with an old-fashioned, authoritative and strict father, and a somewhat rejective mother. Apparently David has always been his mother's favorite, and since his hospitalization he has monopolized the family's attention. This has served to intensify Sam's misbehavior. Bright and imaginative, he has resented his father's authority and his mother's rejection. All his life he has tried to rebel against authority because it represented his father's unpleasant behavior toward him. This accounted in part for his extreme hostility toward policemen, who to him are just another variety of paternal authority. His repeated petty thefts and other minor delinquencies expressed on the one hand his desire for attention, even if it be a criticizing and punishing one, and on the other hand symbolized his rebellion against authority.

On the whole, Sam was friendly and sociable, and if given sufficient attention he will improve substantially. No signs of psychosis or any ideas of persecution were present, but he showed many signs of a neurosis, such as bed wetting, nail biting, temper tantrums and talking in his sleep. It was interesting to note that when asked about his future plans he replied that his greatest wish was to become a policeman. It expressed again his ambivalent attitude toward his father and authority in general. In his personality are also signs of sexual disturbance, more so than is usual in an adolescent of his age and background. He was disturbed about sexual relationships between his parents and seemed very jealous of his father in this area. He had guilt feelings about masturbation, but there was no definite indication of homosexuality, despite the fact that his good looks invited homosexual approaches. Immaturity and illogical reasoning were apparent in his thinking processes.

The examining psychiatrists concluded that Sam had many neurotic traits which could be helped by regular psychotherapy and some understanding and attention from his parents. With a diagnosis of a neurotic character disorder and a hopeful prognosis, they recommended that he be placed on probation and be treated in the Bellevue Mental Hygiene Clinic. The court accepted their advice, but Sam did not do well on probation. He refused to attend the clinic and as soon as he reached 16 he joined the merchant marine.

Prognosis for Sam is guarded, since he is not receptive to treatment.

WILFRED B.

Wilfred, 15½ and a pupil in the 8A grade, is a tall, slender, good-looking boy who could easily pass as two years older than his actual age. He has a cautious, reserved manner, is tense, and seems to be consciously exercising control in an effort to conceal his real feelings. Wilfred has rarely attended school since he was in 1A grade. After prolonged marital friction, Mrs. B. left her husband, an alcoholic, when she realized that their children, Ellen, 16, and Wilfred were frightened by Mr. B.'s incessant abuse. Since then the family has received public assistance. At the time Wilfred was 8 he sent in a false fire alarm resulting in a serious accident, during which a man was killed and three people were injured. Immediately thereafter the school referred Wilfred to the Bureau of Child Guidance because he was in a dazed and disturbed condition. Clinical findings were malnutrition, severe educational retardation in reading, spelling, and arithmetic, despite normal intelligence, and deep anxiety connected with home difficulties, and with scholastic retardation. Wilfred revealed great rivalry between Ellen and himself, which has existed from the time of his earliest memories.

When Wilfred was brought into court for long-standing truancy, he was remanded to a temporary shelter for a short period, and full clinical study was ordered as a guide to the court in attempting to help him. Medical tests showed him to be in good health except for being underweight and having carious teeth. He graded at a 5A level in arithmetic and reading, but achieved an I.Q. of 102 on the Wechsler-Bellevue scale, denoting average intelligence. A diversity of 26 points between his verbal score of 90 and his performance score of 116 was suggestive of strong intellectual dysfunctioning attributable to his educational retardation and emotional disturbance. His fund of general information was poor, while his judgment and reasoning ability were restricted and approximated the upper dull-normal range of intelligence. Wilfred demonstrated good manipulative dexterity as well as ability to organize and synthesize into meaningful wholes. The psychologist noted that Wilfred was subdued throughout the tests and offered no spontaneous comments. While his achievement showed considerable retardation in basic scholastic skills, he could respond to remedial instruction. However, since Wilfred is not interested in school but possesses manual ability, vocational training was recommended for him.

In psychiatric interviews Wilfred was tense, subdued, reserved, and extremely vague and noncommittal in his replies. A confusion of lateral dominance was indicated by the fact that he is right-handed and left-eyed. He revealed more affection for his father than his mother, and feels very badly that his father does not communicate with him and is not interested in him. The psychiatrist was of the opinion that Wilfred is under considerable tension and is very much disturbed by family factors, but he makes a determined effort to conceal the real intensity of his feelings and the true extent of his disturbance. He urgently needs the companionship of a paternal figure, as the abrupt rejection of his father constituted a severe trauma. He feels self-conscious about his height and seeks to compensate for this by associating with older boys and in obtaining jobs by falsifying his age. Wilfred has been unable to establish an adequate, secure relationship with his mother or sister, and the psychiatrist recommended that effort be made to help the mother recognize and provide more fully for his emotional needs in the home. No antisocial tendencies were observed.

Probation was advised and the court followed this recommendation. Referral to a mental hygiene clinic was made, but proved unsuccessful, as Wilfred did not respond to psychiatric treatment. Dental care was provided and Mrs. B. was encouraged to practice better nutrition. There was a slight improvement in attendance. Then Wilfred reached 16 and qualified for an employment certificate, which was granted. He finds much satisfaction in clerking and contributes most of his earnings to his family.

The chances are that Wilfred will be a law-abiding citizen, since he has no antisocial tendencies and manifested no destructive behavior toward people.

ARTHUR D.

Arthur, 14 and enrolled in the second term of high school, is the eldest of three siblings whose mother is a housewife and whose father is a truck driver earning $40 weekly. All during elementary school Arthur earned good marks and his attendance on the whole was satisfactory. Ever since his entrance into high school he has been a habitual truant and was referred to the court on this charge. Although short-tempered, Mrs. D. is warm-hearted, easy-going, and affectionate toward her husband and children. Mr. D., on the other hand, does not find it easy to get along with his family and is inclined to be rigid and punitive. He tries to do what he considers best for his children but finds it difficult to understand the problems of an adolescent boy. Arthur feels exceptionally close to his mother but is confused in his feelings towards his father. Arthur associates with other truants and has been easily influenced by them. They are fond of flying pigeons, loitering in a neighborhood candy store, playing ball in vacant lots, and riding subways. When his father reprimands him for these activities, Arthur leaves home for a few days and sleeps with his grandfather or other relatives. Arthur's late hours have caused violent friction between him and his father.

Before deciding what to do about Arthur, the court remanded him for several weeks to a temporary detention home and ordered clinical study. His adjustment there was not altogether smooth, as in the beginning he was tense and anxious, trying to cloak his fear by belligerent attitudes toward other boys and staff members. Medical findings were negative except for enlarged tonsils and carious teeth. Otherwise Arthur was in good physical condition. On psychometric tests he rated as of low average intelligence with an I.Q. of 91, with marked educational retardation in reading and arithmetic. There was a considerable scatter within the test patterns suggestive of uneven intellectual functioning based partly on emotional factors.

Psychiatric examination showed that Arthur is definitely neurotic, impulsive, and immature for his age. His enuresis, his habit of pulling out his hair, petty thefts, episodes of running away, together with his persistent truancy, beginning almost immediately after the birth of his baby sister, all point toward a neurotic personality. Probation was recommended with transfer to a vocational school and referral to a mental hygiene clinic.

These suggestions the court followed, and as he continued to obtain psychiatric treatment, Arthur's school record became more and more satisfactory. He was discharged from probation after receiving A's in both conduct and attendance.

There is every indication that Arthur has received timely help.

Deep Anxiety

Henry A.

Henry, 12 and a pupil in the 5B grade, is an only child who was born out of wedlock. He has never known his father and his mother's present husband deserted her several years ago. Because of defiant behavior in school, during which he destroyed his books, kicked in a classroom door, and attempted to strike his teacher, Henry was suspended from school and referred to the court. His school record has been marked by frequent truancy and temper outbursts. On his health card are notations of infected scalp, ringworm, colds, diseased tonsils, failure to hear questions, and emotional disturbances. When his retardation in reading and arithmetic became apparent, Henry was given remedial instruction, but this did not help much, due to his absences from class.

Since his temper tantrums are unusually violent, the court remanded Henry to Bellevue Hospital Psychiatric Division for a three-week period of observation. Mrs. A. became so hysterical at the judge's order that she too was sent to Bellevue. Medical findings on both were essentially negative except for many dental caries, which were treated. Psychometric examination of Henry gave him an I.Q. of 103 on the Bellevue scale, denoting average intelligence. A diversity of 30 points between his verbal score of

87 and his performance score of 117 was ascribed to emotional problems and his educational retardation. He rated zero in spelling, 1B in reading, and 3A in arithmetic. Psychiatric observation showed that Henry is anxious and depressed, with a strong dependence upon his mother, who herself was found to be a very neurotic person. He has a deep concern over his lack of a father and over his school difficulties, expressing a marked sense of guilt and inferiority concerning his behavior in class. The psychiatrists concluded that Henry has been infantilized by his mother and is much too dependent upon her. They felt that his disturbance would become even more severe if he were not removed from her care, and they recommended that he be placed in a noncorrectional institution for normal boys of his age group.

The court found it impossible to arrange a placement due to the lack of public facilities and the fact that the only private institutions which had a few vacancies were unwilling to accept him because of his aggressive behavior. As it would be destructive for him to remain out of school, roaming the streets, the court effected his readmission to elementary school.

It is likely that Henry's misconduct will become more and more serious as he grows older, and he probably will then be committed to a state correctional institution. It is a tragedy that a suitable placement is unavailable now when he could be helped to avoid a career of delinquency and crime.

GEORGE N.

George, 13 and in the 6A grade, is the youngest of five siblings whose mother is a widow. He was referred to the court for persistent truancy which he has indulged in since he entered school at the age of 7, four years after his father's death of a heart ailment. The family received public assistance for a period of nine years. George's elder brother is an inmate of a state prison, serving a sentence for robbery. Their eldest sister, a mental defective, gave birth to an illegitimate child after being charged with a sex offense. Alice, the youngest sister, was a habitual truant until she became 16 and secured an employment certificate. Also living in the household is Mrs. N.'s brother, Edward, aged 29 and unemployed, who is a cripple and a former patient in a state mental hospital. George explained his truancy by stating that he likes the "wide open spaces" and hates confinement in classrooms. He associates with known delinquents and recently was arrested with two of them for petty thefts, but was discharged when it was learned that he was already under the jurisdiction of the School Part of the Court.

The court remanded George to Bellevue Hospital Psychiatric Division for observation before deciding how to assist him. Shortly after he had run away from the person escorting him, George was apprehended and taken to a temporary shelter awaiting a bed at Bellevue. In the shelter George exhibited a great deal of anxiety. He habitually held his face down, looking out fearfully from the top of his eyes, and cried that he hated being in a place with doors, a roof, and people. Repeatedly he asked for his mother, crying that he wants her to go with him wherever he goes, and that when he is away from home he does not know what to do and feels lost. At the same time he revealed that he is conflicted in his feeling toward her and often expressed a great deal of hostility toward her and toward himself. For a period he neither slept nor ate and reiterated that he would "have to get out even if I have to kill someone." His panic about closed spaces extends to schools and indeed to any place where he feels that he is not loved. George told the social worker that he has few friends and is so fearful that he claimed never to have been in a fight. He expressed deep feelings of guilt and inferiority, calling himself with considerable emotion "a no-good bum," "a rat," and a "double-crosser." George soon got over his panic at the shelter but was sullen and wanted to retaliate for being kept there when he wanted so badly to go home. All their observations of George led the shelter authorities to conclude that he very much needed psychiatric study.

During his stay at Bellevue, George was found to be in good physical condition except for excessive acne on face and trunk, and a hydrocele. The neurological examination, including an electro-encephalogram, was negative. In psychometric tests George scored an I.Q. of 105, which is high average intelligence. Verbally he rated 95, and on performance 114. The Rorschach test showed a great amount of anxiety, feelings of inadequacy, and some signs of withdrawal and self-punishing tendencies together with a degree of depression and an excellent capacity for identification.

Psychiatric observation bore out these findings. George was seen to be friendly, obedient, quiet, fearful, anxious to please, and always on the verge of pleasing. He is very immature, insecure, and excessively attached to and dependent on his mother. His truancy is pointedly due to his desire to remain at home with her, as it represents the greatest amount of security to him. Outside environment, such as school and neighborhood, causes him fear and anxiety. George has some insight into his condition and is intensely depressed by it. He puts all blame upon himself and reveals many ideas of self-depreciation and self-punishment. He has a number of neurotic habits such as nail biting, bed wetting, nightmares, etc. His acne is a trial to him, for he resents it and feels conspicuous because of it. How far his hydrocele is responsible for his insecurity, especially his sexual insecurity, could not be determined. A diagnosis of anxiety neurosis was made, with a recommendation that he be placed on probation and his mother be advised to encourage George to be out of the house more, to attend school, and to mix more with people. George was accepted for treatment in the Mental Hygiene Clinic of Bellevue Hospital.

Prognosis for George is good as he responds well to treatment.

MANUEL P.

Manuel is 12 years of age and a pupil in the 6B grade. He is the oldest of three siblings whose father is a plasterer and whose mother is a fur operator. The parents leave for work at 8 A.M., send the children to school and return home at 6 P.M. Mr. and Mrs. P. have been known to a mental hygiene clinic for the past six years, where the latter has been a patient diagnosed as a psychoneurotic. Both are described as nervous and irritable. The father has a history of irregular employment, and neither he nor the mother, who recently has complained of head pains and loss of appetite, seems to take much interest in their children. Manuel's younger brother, Jose, has been ill for months with severe pains in his legs and with a high fever, but their parents have apparently been too preoccupied to do much about Jose's illness.

Manuel was brought into court for habitual truancy and for biting a teacher who attempted to prevent his running out of the classroom. The school authorities described him as a behavior problem ever since he entered the first grade, and as a nervous, thin child who is usually twisting his head and biting his nails. Manuel told the court he spends as little time as possible in his home. He likes to play in vacant lots, picking up bottles and scrap. His father stated that Manuel is a bad boy who steals, never stays home, and is always out on the street from early morning until late at night. On the judge's advice, Mr. P. arranged medical care for Jose.

In order that the court might have expert opinion regarding Manuel, based upon twenty-four hour a day observation, he was remanded to Bellevue Hospital Psychiatric Division for a period of three weeks. Medical examination showed that Manuel is well developed and healthy although underweight. He achieved an I.Q. of 95 on the Bellevue intelligence scale, with a verbal score of 102 and a performance score of 89. On educational tests some retardation was evident, with a rating of 6A in spelling, 4B in arithmetic, and 4B to 5A in reading. He was classified as having average intelligence and his scholastic retardation was ascribed to his bilingual home, emotional disturbance and infrequent school attendance.

Observation on the ward revealed that Manuel is an insecure, restless, and dissatisfied neurotic child who has a history of neurotic traits since early childhood, with periods of bed wetting and soiling, poor eating habits and numerous complaints of non-existent illnesses. His mother's hypochondriacal and neurotic tendencies have inclined her to encourage rather than discourage him in these mechanisms. In psychiatric interviews Manuel is inclined to be anxious, irritable, to elaborate his own anxiety dreams, his psychosomatic complaints and to boast of his unstable behavior, but whenever possible shifting responsibility to others. He expressed a feeling that his father is unsympathetic and prefers Jose. In summary, the examining psychiatrists stated that Manuel is a boy whose constitutional endowment is adequate for normal development, his physical condition is generally satisfactory, and his behavior is attributable to neurotic traits. He is in need of a better routinized life with socializing activities and would benefit from placement in a training school. His neurotic traits are reactions to his neurotic parents and the emotionally disturbed home life.

Acting upon this advice, the court tried first to place Manuel in a private rehabilitative institution but when no vacancy was available and his misconduct became more flagrant, he was committed to a state correctional institution. Their report stated that Manuel is receiving psychiatric treatment and is making a fair adjustment to a stable routine.

Prognosis for Manuel seems guarded because his destructive home life has affected him so adversely and it may be that despite the stable routine in a state correctional institution other elements there, such as association with older, more confirmed delinquents, will serve to increase his negative patterns.

FRANK E.

Frank, 11 and a student in the 5A grade, has a sister, 14, and two brothers, 9 and 4. All these children are unhappy and fearful and have lived first with both parents, then alternately with their mother, paternal relatives, maternal relatives, in orphanages, and currently with their father. When brought into court for excessive truancy, Frank was residing with his mother. Both parents are extremely unstable and rejective of their children, while the marital relationship has been destructive from the start. Mr. E. was abusive and violent toward his wife and children, gambled, drank heavily, and deserted frequently. Records show that he had had six admissions to a local psychiatric hospital within a three-year period, and in this process a great deal of individual and family psychopathology and disharmony had been disclosed. Diagnoses made for him were psychopathic personality with psychotic episodes. He himself had had a most unsatisfying childhood. Both of his parents were abusive and unsocial, especially his father. On Mr. E.'s last admission he was under an order of Magistrates' Court for writing threatening letters to his wife, and the hospital reported to that court:

"He is not a mere crank or tyrant in the home, but has the morbidly heightened egocentricity of a person suffering from a paranoid type of mental illness, and if there were not a wife to threaten, his dangerous tendencies would have found other expressions."

Mr. E. told the hospital authorities that he had been opposed to the birth of his children, and when Frank was an infant Mr. E. threatened to kill the boy. At the conclusion of his sixth admission to a psychopathic ward, Mr. E. was committed to a state hospital for the mentally ill where he remained a year and then escaped into another state. He and Mrs. E. have not maintained a home together since his commitment.

Mrs. E. is an extremely difficult person, antagonistic and distrustful of all forms of authority. She was employed intermittently as a restaurant worker, receiving public relief when remaining at home with her children. She resented their presence, sending them to relatives when she preferred to be by herself and work.

When Frank was 9, school authorities referred him to a guidance unit because he was withdrawn, unduly restless, inattentive, stubborn, and failing in all his subjects. It was at this time that his father was committed to a state institution. In response to an inquiry his mother told the clinic that Frank had had convulsive seizures beginning at $1\frac{1}{2}$, after having been knocked down by another child, and ending at 6 following an automobile accident. Ever since the second episode he has stuttered. He has stolen and set fires in hallways. From the time he was an infant he has feared and dreaded his father. When truanting he sat home reading comics or wandered about on the streets. He was found to be functioning on a dull normal level with good perception and planning on performance tests. He complained of nightmares, had difficulty in expressing himself, and his general maladjustment seemed severe.

Much against Mrs. E.'s will, the judge ordered that Frank be studied in the court's clinic. Physically he was found to be in good condition. In psychometric tests he had an I.Q. of 82, which was felt to be unrepresentative of his innate ability due to malfunctioning. It was hard for him to think; he sat frowning, tearing at a blotter with head hanging down, wringing his hands. Scholastically he was greatly retarded, doing fourth-grade arithmetic and being unable to read. During psychiatric examination Frank was withdrawn, staring into space, then tense and angry, with facial grimaces and mild mannerisms. When asked for his father's whereabouts, Frank replied "in jail," then immediately corrected this to "in the army." He was so unresponsive that the psychiatrist could not establish a relationship with him, and since the possibility of organic brain disease could not be ruled out, the clinic recommended that Frank be sent to Bellevue Hospital Psychiatric Division for a period of observation.

Despite vigorous opposition from Mrs. E., the court followed the clinic's advice and remanded Frank to Bellevue for a period of three weeks. There the physical findings were confirmed, but he scored a much higher I.Q.—101, with a performance rating of 117 and a verbal of 85. The lower verbal functioning was attributed partly to severe emotional problems and blocking in these fields and partly to his reading disability, accounting partially for his truancy. Experience indicates that children who show this particular stubborn type of refusal to attend school usually have a deep-seated emotional problem connected with the family condition, with resulting anxiety. Neurological examinations ruled out the possibility of a brain disorder. Psychiatric observations disclosed that Frank was disturbed but not given to open aggression or temper tantrums, although antagonistic to routine and especially hostile to psychiatric interviews, during which he became stubborn, sullen, noncommunicative, and under pressure cried and ran out of the room. He was never happy but, instead, was usually irritable and preoccupied. Hospital authorities attempted an intensive program of psychotherapy for Frank in an effort to help him express his problems and come to some understanding of these. Play therapy, group activities, drugs (sodium amytal), hypnotherapy, fostering a relationship with one therapist were all tried, but very limited success was achieved, because these attempts were interfered with repeatedly by his mother's visits. She encouraged him in a negative attitude toward the hospital, schools, courts and his father. Frank loosened up to a slight extent and was able to express his unhappiness and conflicts concerning his father but was unable to express his difficulties regarding his mother, which appeared even more profound. The psychiatrists felt that Frank has never known any positive experiences in his life. Whatever relationships he has had with his parents have been negative and destructive. So far he has never had any security.

It was concluded that he has an above-average constitutional endowment but was suffering from a severe distortion in personality development as a result of his unhappy life experiences, intensified by his inability to read, which further blocked his school adjustment and his capacity for expressing himself. He was not mentally ill, the diagnosis being: anxiety state in a boy of good potentialities, handicapped by a pronounced reading disability.

Bellevue therefore recommended that Frank be placed in an institution for normal boys with a program of socializing activities, remedial instruction, and psychiatric help to gain insight into his problems once a separation from his mother is accomplished.

At the expiration of the remand period, Frank was returned to court accompanied by his mother. As soon as placement was broached, she became very upset and refused to consider it. Moved by her pleas, the court paroled the boy to her while a search for a suitable placement was made. When one was found Mrs. E. and Frank were summoned to court, but they did not appear and it was later learned that she had left the state, sending all her children to their father in Maryland.

Continuing in a life of insecurity and chaotic parental behavior throughout his formative years, Frank's personality undoubtedly will become more disordered. It is sad that he was not placed in a temporary shelter pending placement at the expiration of the remand to Bellevue, for it was obvious that his mother would not consent to placement.

MILDRED R.

Mildred, 15 and in the first term of high school, is the eldest of five siblings whose father died when she was 12. Their mother is employed part time as a saleswoman and works hard to keep the home clean and attractive. She was worried at finding several checks which Mildred had taken from a concern where she had worked during the summer vacation. On two occasions when money disappeared, it was thought that Mildred had stolen it, so she was discharged. Since she first entered school Mildred had been a persistent truant, using her daily lunch money for movies and subway rides. During the last semester she did not appear for any test, weekly, monthly, mid-term, or end of term, and therefore received no grades. When she receives permission to remain out until 11 P.M., she does not return until 3 or 4 A.M. and refuses to give any account of her activities. On her health card impaired vision and flat feet were noted.

When Mildred was referred to the court for habitual truancy, she appeared very disturbed and distraught. The judge thereupon remanded her to Bellevue Hospital Psychiatric Division for a period of observation. Aside from a lacerated hymen the medical findings were negative, although she has been physically ill since early childhood and has spent the greater part of her life in hospitals suffering from osteomyelitis and other infections. Psychometric tests disclosed that Mildred has average intelligence, with an I.Q. of 100 on the Bellevue scale. Poor performance on digits was the only outstanding deviation in her test patterns, and this suggested emotional disturbance and preoccupation. Her reasoning ability is good but her work habits are of low quality. She adjusted slowly to each test, asking many unnecessary questions. The Rorschach pattern revealed a highly disturbed and anxious girl whose familial relationships are a source of deep worry to her.

Psychiatric observation indicated that Mildred's long periods of physical illness and hospitalization have made her feel different from other children and have estranged her from her younger siblings. Another severe trauma was the death of her father while she was in a hospital at a critical psychological stage in her life. One of her major problems is her feeling of rejection by her mother, whose love and affection she craves. Although she admires her mother very much, the fact that she is young and attractive causes Mildred to feel jealous and she expressed her jealousy in temper outbursts, and disobedient behavior. She resents her mother's preference for John, the youngest sibling. Mildred has some insight concerning her difficulties and is eager to be helped. The examining psychiatrists were of the opinion that Mildred is suffering from deep anxiety and a neurotic conduct disorder requiring intensive psychotherapy. Considering her home conditions, they felt she would make a far better adjustment while living elsewhere and therefore recommended placement in a private institution having psychiatric facilities.

Their advice was followed by the court, and Mildred has made substantial progress. She obtains satisfaction from her mother's regular visits and seems more willing to share in her mother's affections.

Schizoid Features

In the two cases that follow there are schizoid features denoting very serious emotional disturbance. Both children apparently need care which they are unable to obtain in their own homes.

ARNOLD W.

Arnold, 14 and a pupil in the 7A grade, was brought into court for excessive truancy. He is the eldest of five children whose father is a tugboat captain and is twenty-one years older than his wife. Mr. W. spends very little time in the home, which is dirty and dilapidated. Mrs. W., obese and strong looking, suffers from a kidney condition and high blood pressure. She contends that she has to sit or lie down during the day and cannot look after the home or her children. She seems to enjoy ill health, relating with gusto the details of her hospitalizations. On Arnold's health card are noted frequent headaches, exhaustion, poor sleep habits, bad posture, excessive use of the lavatory, and coughing spells. At the age of six he had a bowel resection performed. He is large and athletic looking, an excellent swimmer, and enjoys basketball and stick ball.

To aid the court in attempting to help Arnold the judge ordered medical, psychometric, and psychiatric study in a mental hygiene clinic. Arnold was accompanied by his mother, who talked quite frankly with the psychiatrist. She appeared to be immature, inadequate, unreliable, very bland and superficial, with no insight into the seriousness of the parental lack of supervision in the home. She disclosed that both she and her husband are chronic alcoholics who care little about their children.

Medical findings for Arnold were essentially negative. On psychological tests—Stanford-Binet and Bellevue adult scale—he scored an I.Q. of 118 and was classed as of high average intelligence. In psychiatric interviews he was seen to be insecure, withdrawn, tense, and blocked due to emotional obstruction and self-absorption. He leads a rich phantasy life and neglects practical requirements. Infantile sexual trends were evinced with an unwholesome fantasy attachment to his mother. His position of eldest child and being "the man of the house" fosters his confusion. Schizoid feaures are evident in his development which require periodic check throughout his adolescent period. He is too self-preoccupied to concentrate on academic subjects. A psychiatric classification was made of primary behavior disorder with schizoid feaures, with a recommendation for placement and manual training.

Acting upon this advice, the judge committed Arnold to an excellent rehabilitative institution for boys of his age group. Their report stated that his schizoid patterns are becoming more pronounced. It is feared that he is likely to become mentally ill.

Prognosis for Arnold is poor, due to his deteriorating emotional balance. In our present state of knowledge, his eventual mental illness appears almost inevitable.

BILL D.

Bill is a very unhappy boy who was 14 and in 7B grade when he was first brought into the court for habitual truancy during the last three years. He is the youngest of seven children who live with their mother, a widow, whose husband died when Bill was 2. Mrs. D. has tried to cooperate with school authorities, but at times Bill is beyond her control. Often he rides the subways all night long and recently was apprehended by a truant officer while working for a newspaper delivery truck late at night. Once he was seen helping a motorman drive a trolley at 2 A.M. Bill likes to "hang around" bus terminals and seems fascinated by any type of transportation. He is not defiant to his mother but shows rivalry and resentment toward his next oldest sibling, Agnes. Mrs. D. attributes Bill's truancy to an insatiable wanderlust and a desire to work.

First the court scheduled a psychological examination for Bill when it appeared that he might be mentally retarded. A Rorschach test was included to see if emotional disturbance might also be a factor in his behavior. Bill scored an I.Q. of 69 on the Bellevue-Wechsler test, rating in the retarded range on general intelligence. A marked reading disability was noted. The Rorschach pattern was that of an extremely disturbed boy with schizoid features, whereupon psychiatric study was recommended. Mrs. D. was opposed to this, expressing a feeling that there was nothing whatever the matter with Bill and pleading with the judge to just let Bill return to school. After full discussion the judge ordered that Bill be examined in the court clinic.

There he was found to be much overgrown for his age, with

carious teeth and a slight internal strabismus of the left eye.
Neurological tests showed tremors of the tongue and hands, fair
coordination but sluggish reflexes. On the Stanford-Binet scale
Bill achieved an I.Q. of 80. He had great difficulty in expressing
himself verbally and became confused in his explanations. Slight
traces of a speech defect were present. On the Stenquist scale he
was equaled or exceeded by only 38 per cent of 15 year old boys,
indicating fair manual ability. The examiner recommended that
his future training should be entirely along mechanical lines. In
psychiatric interviews Bill gave the impression of being a disturbed child with a schizoid make-up. From the history which the
mother gave and from observation of the child, the psychiatrist
felt that Bill might have an organic involvement of the brain. An
electro-encephalogram would be helpful in clearing the diagnosis.
The clinic therefore recommended that Bill be observed in the
Psychiatric Division of Bellevue Hospital for a period of two or
three weeks.

Upon learning of this proposal Mrs. D., vehemently opposed it,
although she herself was at a loss to deal with Bill whose truancy
and nightly escapades continued. She offered to have him studied
by a private psychiatrist, and the court accepted her plan. Bill
kept several appointments with this psychiatrist and then ceased.
There has been no improvement in Bill's conduct. It is questionable whether he will be accessible to treatment while remaining at
home. Mrs. D. now feels he needs placement and keeps trying to
arrange for his admission to a private school. She fears that while
on one of his nightly journeys Bill might become involved with
adult delinquents. But private schools for boys like Bill are few
and highly expensive. In the meantime, the court has no placement available for Bill.

It is likely that Bill will soon be participating in serious
delinquency, for he cannot seem to control his wayward impulses and his mental retardation renders him a prey to older,
more intelligent delinquents.

Psychoneurotic Patterns

ERNEST L.

Ernest was referred to the court for excessive school absence. Nine years old and in 2A grade, he cries at the mention of school and becomes hysterical whenever efforts are made to force his attendance. At the age of 4 he was first entered in school, spent one day in class and then was removed by his parents. He was brought back one year later and, again, immediately withdrawn. This process was repeated the following year, and because he was still under 7 he was discharged as being under compulsory school age. Then he reappeared at 8 and was admitted to the 1B grade, although chronologically he was retarded three terms. He attended thirty-five days, due chiefly to the fact that the truant officer bodily placed him in class. At the end of the semester he was placed in the 2A grade even though his achievement did not warrant it.

From the Attendance Bureau it was learned that Ernest is very dependent upon and overindulged by his mother. He spends most of his time at home and does not enjoy playing with other children; apparently he has been unable to develop normal group attachments. When these matters were brought to the court's attention, it was decided to have Ernest studied at the Bureau of Child Guidance of the Board of Education. Their study was delayed by broken appointments due to the parents' ill health.

It was found that Ernest has low average intelligence, with an I.Q. of 90, and that his refusal to attend school is based on a severe psychoneurosis of childhood. He actually is deeply frightened when in school, which is a place of dread and horror to him. It was therefore recommended that no further efforts be made to force his attendance until after he has received psychiatric help. Ernest's serious emotional disturbance is ascribed to his home conditions. He is the eighth of ten living children and was born after the death of an 18 months old child when his mother was extremely upset over her loss. She has been nervous and ill ever since that time. Both parents, especially the mother, have used unwise methods in handling Ernest. She weeps easily, complains constantly of her pains and discomfort, and tells him that he makes her ill. She understands no way of disciplining him except yelling, screaming, and striking. When she beats him both become exceedingly upset and weep together. Ernest has learned that crying and emotional outbursts will get him what he wants and is not averse to using these tools often. While he has the intelligence to progress normally in school, his emotional disturbance is such that he is far behind in his studies and will need remedial instruction when he is able to go to school. It is significant that he has not yet learned to read or do simple arithmetic.

The psychiatrist concluded that Ernest is badly in need of psychiatric treatment and that it is equally important for his parents to be given an understanding of better ways to handle him. Treatment of both Ernest and his parents can be accomplished only gradually and during this period he should be exempted from school. Accepting the advice of the clinic, the court arranged for Ernest to be excused from school while he and his parents were receiving psychiatric assistance in a mental hygiene clinic and until in the opinion of the clinic Ernest would be ready for school.

It seems a pity that the school authorities did not deal adequately with this case within their own facilities. Surely it was not necessary for Ernest and his parents to be brought into court when the same type of study could have been arranged in the same clinic by the principal, and the assistant superintendent could have excused Ernest from attendance while undergoing treatment. The court's authority need not be evoked for such action. It is to be hoped that similar problems will be acted upon without referral to courts. The situation would be different if the parents after thorough discussion refused help for their child and themselves.

JOSEPH C.

Joseph, 14 and in the first term of a school of industrial art, was brought into court on a charge of habitual truancy. He is the only child of his parents' second marriage and has three adult stepsiblings, a stepbrother, and two stepsisters, all of whom now have their own homes. Mr. C., a carpenter, earns about $40 weekly; Mrs. C. busies herself in the household. Previously Joseph had been referred to a guidance clinic by his older married stepsister who had received counseling service from the same agency. She described Joe as high-strung, nervous, and given to severe temper tantrums. Several times he had run away from home.

The clinic found Mrs. C. to be a very rigid, exacting, and dominating person who controls each situation in the home by her compulsive rigidity or by exploiting her illness. She has subjected all the members of the household to a highly restrictive and prohibitive home environment from which the children have striven in various ways to escape. Joseph's two stepsisters were in difficulties as a reaction to their oppressive home atmosphere. Mr. C. is ineffectual and completely submissive to his wife. He has never been able to protect any of the children from her demands. Joseph was seen at the clinic on an intensive psychotherapeutic basis. He complained of frequent bad headaches which, he said, he had had as long as he could remember. He tires easily, is anxious in a new situation, perspiring very freely with no apparent provocation. Responding to the psychiatric social worker, Joseph established a good relationship with him and brought out many of his fears and anxieties. While there was some progress, he continued to truant and ran away from home six times, remaining away from one to six days. He told of spending all of his time during these periods riding the subways day and night.

Joseph's truancy was felt to be a reaction against his mother's nagging, rigidity, and destructive behavior. His greatest tie is to his father, with whom he identifies and sympathizes. He resists his father's submissiveness to his mother and finds it painful to observe. Each summer Joseph has been sent to camp he made an excellent adjustment, enjoying his stay and pleading to remain longer, with regret for the necessity of returning home. It is interesting to note that while at home Joseph has no recreational or social contacts and refused attempts to place him in group activities, describing himself as a "lone wolf." He was also unable to accept the Big Brothers offered him on a friendly, supportive level. Family members reported that he was stealing sums of money from them including, $50 from his mother. He admitted these thefts with an explanation that his parents gave him no spending money. When school reopened, the clinic gave him a weekly allowance of $2 out of a scholarship fund.

On psychometric tests Joseph scored an I.Q. of 121, indicating superior general intelligence. After psychiatric conferences, a diagnosis was made of psychoneurosis, anxiety hysteria, with conduct and habit disorders. Placement in a rehabilitative center was recommended where Joseph could receive continued psychotherapy. In the psychiatrist's opinion Joseph's home environment is so destructive that he cannot cope with it. Joseph willingly accepted the placement effected by the court, for which he had been prepared by intensive study and counseling in the guidance agency. Reports received from the institution state that Joseph is making a splendid adjustment to the group and is responding well to a program of psychiatric treatment.

Prognosis for Joseph is good, as he is receptive to the excellent treatment he is receiving.

CARL W.

Carl, almost 16 and in 8A grade, is both unusually tall for his age and immature. Because of misconduct in class, such as creating disturbances by shouting, clowning, and refusing to do his work, coupled with persistent truancy, he was referred to the court. He is the third youngest of nine children. Two of his older brothers developed mental illnesses; one later committed suicide and the other became a patient in a state hospital, suffering from paranoia. Mr. and Mrs. W. expressed indifference about Carl's school attendance. They let him go his own way. At one time Mr. W. was an inmate of a state hospital for the mentally ill with a diagnosis of manic-depressive psychosis. He often becomes intoxicated on homemade wine and his children tease him about his many food phobias. Actually he has little contact with his family. There is frequent quarreling and incessant friction among members of the household. About a year previously Carl ran away on two occasions to avoid school but returned home of his own volition after several days of absence. With the connivance of his parents, Carl recently tried to join the merchant marine by falsifying his age.

After studying this data the judge remanded Carl to a temporary shelter and ordered medical, psychometric, and psychiatric examinations to be performed at the shelter. He was found to be in good health physically, in fact better developed than most boys of his age. Psychologically, he tested dull normal with an I.Q. of 87 on the Bellevue-Wechsler scale. There was a marked difference of 25 points between his verbal and performance scores, indicating a severe intellectual dysfunctioning due in part to serious emotional insecurity as well as to educational retardation. Analysis of the subtests disclosed rather sharp cleavage between skills on the verbal level, which were essentially of a borderline to low dull normal range, and skills on the performance level which were of average range. Carl demonstrated a poverty of general information, together with restriction in anything pertaining to situations which he has to deal with verbally. On educational tests he gave evidence of marked retardation in both reading and arithmetic, attaining a 5B score. A scholastic program heavily weighted in favor of manual training was recommended for Carl by the psychologist.

Psychiatric observation of Carl and his parents convinced the examiner that all three are very seriously disturbed people. The mother revealed that before her marriage she was advised to enter a mental hospital but she refused and the matter was dropped. She is the dominant member of the household and is rigid in her attitudes. She controls the family finances; one of the topics of fierce arguments between Carl and his mother is money. She is extremely emotional and when faced with difficult problems feels helpless and screams. She frequently tells Carl that she fears he will become insane like his two brothers. Mr. W. impressed the psychiatrist as withdrawn and seclusive.

Carl described a number of symptoms, some neurotic and others suggestive of possible latent psychotic process. When he hears people laughing he believes they are laughing at him. He feels that he is hated by other members of his family because of the arguments he starts and thinks that they tamper with his clothing and other possessions while he sleeps so as to frighten him. Whenever he hears thunder he develops an acute attack of anxiety. Oftentimes he fears he is going insane like his brothers. Carl expressed an obsessional fear of operations and lives in continual dread that the next day he may develop appendicitis. In regard to attacks upon him by other boys, Carl remarked that he had provoked these by squeezing their arms to prove his strength.

On the basis of his observations the psychiatrist concluded that Carl presents a serious emotional disturbance which appears to be in very large part on a psychoneurotic basis. He is extremely immature in his approach to and in his conception of situations and is therefore unable to utilize the mature, volitional discrimination which would ordinarily be expected of boys in his age group. His neurotic fears seem attributable to his emotional experiences in the home and also to his self-consciousness of his tall stature. While having considerable latent aggressive tendencies, he is extremely fearful of these, for they represent the threat of insanity to him. The fact that most of his fears have no factual foundation is somewhat apparent to him; he asked whether he might be helped to overcome these. Carl needs intensive psychiatric treatment. Although his ideas of persecution are vaguely expressed and not well formulated, the possibility of a latent or incipient psychosis must be considered.

Upon receiving these findings, the court arranged for Carl to attend a psychiatric clinic. He keeps his apointments there, is showing slight but steady progress and is no longer such a problem in school.

Prognosis for Carl seems guarded, due to the possibility of his developing a psychosis.

MARK H.

Mark, 15 and in the first term of high school, appears very lonely and depressed. He is the eldest of five children, three of whom are in a private child-caring institution; the fourth child is in a foster home. Mark himself has been in three different orphanages, from each of which he has run away. Only rarely and for brief intervals between separations due to intense marital friction have their parents maintained a home. Mr. H. is a welder and Mrs. H. supports herself as a barmaid. He resides in a furnished room with successive women friends, while she does likewise with men friends.

Since his most recent escape from institutional life, Mark has slept at times in a furnished room adjacent to his mother's or father's room. When he did not attend school over a long period, an intensive search was instituted for Mark by juvenile authorities. He was found to have attached himself to various male adults, being supported and housed by them for weeks or months at a time. Occasionally he did household chores for those who had apartments. He made their acquaintance on the street, in cheap restaurants, or in pool halls, representing himself as a boy without a family and with no one to whom to turn. When he was brought into court for habitual truancy, Mark told the judge, with apparent deep sincerity, that all of the time he was not in school he was employed on a farm in upstate New York earning his maintenance. Not even when the facts of his stay in the city were mentioned to him did he admit the truth.

While undergoing study at the court clinic, Mark was remanded to a temporary shelter. Medically he was found to be undernourished and undersized. In psychometric tests he rated as average, with an I.Q. of 95. The test pattern pointed to a definite intellectual dysfunction on a severe emotional basis. He did not function up to his actual intellectual base and, therefore, the psychometric picture was not a true index of his ability. A strong emotional depression was reflected in his forcing himself to perform the tasks set. The psychologist was of the opinion that basically Mark has the intelligence to complete a high school education and to benefit from a course of study, but it would be impossible for him to do so without intensive psychotherapy.

In psychiatric interviews Mark was seen to be deeply depressed, defensive, vague, and evasive in all matters pertaining to his relationships with his parents and his activities. A confusion of lateral dominance was indicated by the fact that he is left-handed and right-eyed. No evidence of a psychosis or mental defectiveness was present. His scholastic retardation was clearly caused by severe emotional disturbance in psychoneurotic patterns of anxiety and depression. Mark is resentful of authority and supervision as a result of subjection to rigid discipline in a child-caring institution of the old-fashioned type. He reiterated a desire to have his parents reunited and the children together with them. He prefers his mother to his father but is reticent about this. As a result of neurotic anxiety, Mark has a compulsive drive to be with his mother and his behavior is characterized by a strong degree of immaturity, impulsiveness, and hostility toward authority. Because of his seriously disturbed personality and the lack of a suitable home, placement was imperative for Mark. The psychiatrist therefore recommended that Mark be placed in a controlled environment where he could receive intensive psychotherapy.

No private rehabilitative institution was willing to accept Mark because of his long history of running away, and no public institution for him existed except a correctional one. The court had no alternative but to commit him to the latter.

It is feared that Mark will come out several years hence even more embittered and probably definitely antisocial. His misbehavior seems due to neglect—neglect on the part of his parents and society.

NEIL R.

Neil, 10 years of age and in the 2B grade, was referred to the court after suspension from school for sadistic aggression toward other children. He is a frail, unhappy boy who had been brought into another division of the court the previous year for assaults on fellow pupils and had been remanded twice to Bellevue Hospital Psychiatric Division for observation. Placement had been suggested but could not be effected due to lack of facilities. Neil is an only child whose mother has been diagnosed as psychoneurotic. Teachers reported that he was always hurting other children or destroying their handiwork. He punched them in the stomach, put pins in their backs, twisted their arms, threw missiles about the room trying to hurt them, bullied them, and on one occasion he struck a child in the eye with a baseball bat and hospital care was required. He often truanted, remained out late at night, sometimes all night, and seemed entirely beyond his parents' control.

At the first Bellevue remand, Neil revealed deep anxiety and frequent impulsive aggression toward other children, keeping the ward routine in a turmoil. When his mother came to take him home he refused to go with her and she removed him by force. She evinced considerable emotional instability and obsessive attitudes toward Neil's toilet training and habits. Both parents were described as very much on the defensive, distrustful, critical, and always encouraging Neil in the feeling that he was abused in the hospital, stating in his presence that they would "expose" the hospital in newspaper publicity or appeal to political influence. In the psychiatrists' opinion Neil is a child whose constitutional endowment is about average, who shows a psychoneurotic reaction to a neurotic, disturbed mother and a less seriously disturbed father. Neil has not succeeded in making any normal social adjustment at school or outside the home. If he is to be returned home, his mother should receive psychiatric care and guidance. A more sound program would be his temporary placement in an institution from which he cannot escape for a period of training and psychotherapy. Since the initial period of consistent observation in the ward had been brief and disturbed by the parents, the hospital requested that the court send Neil back for further observation and psychotherapy prior to placement, provided the parents accepted this plan.

Immediately thereafter he was returned to Bellevue by the court with an admonition to his mother not to disturb him there. He was defiant and difficult during this remand period, taking part in antisocial behavior with other children. The conclusion reached was that since Neil was in the middle of a psychotherapeutic process, he should be returned to the hospital for another month of continued intensive psychotherapy preparatory to placement. As the parents protested this strenuously, he was placed on probation pending a placement which did not materialize.

When Neil's conduct became progressively worse, he was suspended and the present referral to court was made. When his parents were interviewed separately they divulged their growing anxiety about Neil, who has taken to remaining away from home for several days and nights at a time with no coherent explanation of his whereabouts or activities. Mr. R. also spoke of his fears that his wife is becoming mentally ill. He has urged her to seek psychiatric help, but she is adamant in her refusal. Both of them realize that her influence on Neil is destructive, but they are at a loss as to what to do. They promised they would do their utmost not to interfere with the court's plan to remand Neil back to Bellevue for further observation and would try to cooperate with the hospital authorities. The court recognized that the parents, as well as Neil, have great difficulty in controlling their impulses.

Findings similar to those in the previous remand periods were reported to the court. Physically Neil is in good condition except for being underweight. On the Bellevue intelligence scale he scored an I.Q. of 94. There were several slight features of an organic type such as confusion in the block design and an inferior Goodenough, but these were traced to his serious emotional disturbance. In educational tests Neil did 2A spelling, reading, and arithmetic. His Rorschach pattern showed a great deal of anxiety and

difficulties in personal relationships and confusion of social attitudes. Neil classified as a boy of average intelligence with severe scholastic retardation related to his psychoneurotic problems.
Observation on the ward showed that Neil's highly disturbed behavior had become intensified. He is never willing to follow the routine of other children and seems totally incapable of identifying himself with children or entering into a classroom situation and settling down to work. Instead he races up and down the halls, striking at children right and left, and shows belligerent, antagonistic behavior toward adults. His present behavior appears less anxious but more antagonistic, perhaps because he has now spent almost two years in successfully defying all plans for his making a regular school adjustment and has not been helped by his parents nor by any other authority in accepting a schedule.

In psychiatric interviews he first avoids and seems incapable of facing any of his problems or of assuming responsibility for his actions. Under pressure he is utterly indignant and angry when asked to admit that he has hit other children, stolen, run away from home, or omitted to do his school work. This attitude has been engendered by his parents' attitudes and by the long period of failure to find a suitable placement for him. When his fantasy life, his dreams, and fears are discussed with him, he reveals an enormous anxiety over his family, particularly his mother. He fears that something will happen to her or that she will leave him. There was added evidence that his family situation is pathological. Neil seemed to be a panicky boy who builds up defenses to protect himself from facing growing up, from escaping from home conditions, and from adapting himself to school and society.

It was the conclusion of the psychiatrists that Neil is of average endowment but suffering from an anxiety psychoneurosis, secondary to a home situation which has become increasingly difficult through the failure to get him placed where he would have normal daily living for a boy of his age. In their opinion there were two choices (1) placing him in an institution with a socializing routine carefully supervised, intense in its program with remedial instruction, and where he could not escape easily, (2) placing him in the children's division of a state hospital for the mentally ill which does not have educational facilities adequate for Neil and where the other children would not offer him sufficient opportunities for socialization, identification, and competition. Furthermore, his entrance into the state hospital would be contingent upon one parent signing admission papers, and this was very unlikely.

Unfortunately, the court was unable to follow the psychiatrists' advice, because no public institution of that nature exists. In New York, the private institutions which had vacancies were unwilling to accept Neil because of his extremely aggressive conduct. Neither parent was willing to sign for his admission to a state hospital, and the educational authorities were disinclined to readmit him to school since he is a menace to other children. As a result, the court is helpless to aid Neil, whose behavior is becoming progressively worse.

The chances are that Neil will be committed to a state hospital for the mentally ill when he seriously injures another child or one of his parents becomes willing for voluntary commitment. It is not sound to force a commitment now when the psychiatrists themselves do not favor a state hospital admission for Neil.

CHAPTER V

PSYCHOPATHIC PERSONALITIES AND THE MENTALLY ILL

IN THIS CHAPTER are examples of youthful offenders who were diagnosed as psychopathic personalities and those who are mentally ill.

PSYCHOPATHIC PERSONALITIES

A stimulating and concrete picture of the psychopath based upon intensive experience has been given by Dr. M. J. Pescor [1] of the Medical Center for Federal Prisoners at Springfield, Missouri. The psychopath is neither psychotic, neurotic, nor feeble-minded in the usual meaning of these words, although he may be mentally retarded as well as psychopathic. These individuals are antisocial, selfish to the extreme, habitually dissatisfied, and restless. Some are characterized as homosexuals and sex perverts. They have no feelings of guilt when they steal, lie, cheat, or engage in other reprehensible conduct. Their antisocial attitudes find early expression in truancy, running away from home, petty thefts. As they reach adulthood, their misconduct becomes progressively worse. To them the mechanism of projection is a ready tool, and since they do not accept any blame for their actions, they continue on their way, not profiting from experience, regardless of punishment. In them social intelligence is lacking and, as a consequence, they are perpetually at odds with other people.

[1] *The Psychopath,* Federal Probation, Vol. IX, No. 1, January-March, 1945, pp. 28-32.

Admittedly the term is broad and is sometimes used cursorily and as a catchall, yet a diagnosis of psychopathic personality should be derived from full medical, psychometric, and psychiatric study. Although there are no psychological tests for social intelligence comparable to tests for other types of intelligence and aptitudes, nevertheless, as Dr. Pescor points out, both the Rorschach test and the electro-encephalograph have diagnostic value in this regard; studies have disclosed that a high proportion of psychopaths show abnormal brain wave patterns.[2] Lack of social intelligence may be inherited or acquired.[3] It may be the result of disease or of birth injuries affecting the brain. As an example of acquired psychopathology, the conduct disturbances of children who were victims of encephalitis were cited. Many students of the problem feel that with our present knowledge there is no successful treatment for psychopathic personalities except segregation. The community needs protection from them and they need to be protected from themselves. Even in correctional institutions they have to be kept apart from the other inmates because of assaultive and destructive behavior. Some of our most vicious criminals belong to this group.

On the other hand, results of a New York project in 1943 under the auspices of the College of Physicians and Surgeons of Columbia University are more encouraging.[4] Prolonged observation revealed elements not readily ascertainable in clinic study. It was shown that persons diagnosed as having psychopathic personalities can be helped to attain some stability by means of medical, laboratory, psychological, and psychiatric examinations, coupled with frequent therapeutic interviews and other specialized treatment. It appeared that

[2] *Ibid.*, p. 30.
[3] *Ibid.;* see also A. J. Rosanoff, *Manual of Psychiatry*, 7th ed. New York, John Wiley & Sons, 1938, pp. 612-642, 651, 652.
[4] Robert Seliger, Edwin Lukas, and Robert Lindner, *Contemporary Criminal Hygiene*. Baltimore, Oakridge Press, 1946, p. 48.

under suitable management, long-time care and supervision, they are not so resistive to treatment as it has been commonly thought. Emotional deprivation was found to be a causal factor, traumatizing experiences scarring the personality very early in its development.[5]

In the following cases early symptoms of psychopathic personality were readily discernible. If adequate help could be made available when these early indications are manifested, much adult delinquency could be prevented, but to date there seems to be very little successful treatment for these children. It is significant that a high degree of parental disorganization and instability is found in the illustrations given.

ALBERT C.

Albert was 15 and a pupil in the first term of high school when he was brought into court because of absences caused by his suspension for misconduct involving suspected abnormal sexuality. For the past three years Albert had been an increasingly serious behavior problem to his teachers, who said of him:

"An evil influence—does not belong in a school where there are girls. Marked tendency toward sexual perversion. Discusses home affairs with fellow pupils. Petition brought to principal by boys in Albert's class asking to have him removed from the class 'because he is always getting our class into trouble and is always fighting with the children.' Albert is particularly annoying to the girls—tries to kiss them—would always touch or push them when they passed by; at times he cursed the girls. Acts in a superior manner toward his classmates and continually tells them of his superiority and of his scorn of them. Made appointments to meet certain boys in the lavatory. Manner of speech, way of walking, and preening motions led teachers to the conclusion that something was wrong with him. Boys would wait after school to beat him up—he bribed some by paying them. Tried and found guilty twenty-three times during one term by student officers. Is quarrelsome—has kicked boys in line and stepped on girls' feet. Annoys girls by pulling their hairpins and hiding their pocketbooks. One

[5] *Ibid.*, pp. 136-137.

girl's arm was burned as he pushed her against a radiator while she was trying to prevent him from throwing her pocketbook out of a window. Craves attention and is always seeking compliments concerning his personal appearance. Never works well with other children. Displays bad temper during which he uses bad language. Has a suggestive way of speaking. Does not seem to have any physical courage. Does not take orders or follow directions. Worked in short spurts but soon destroyed the little he did. He claimed that when he was in the lavatory one day another boy entered, engaged him in conversation and attempted to force him to perform an act of degeneracy. Upon questioning, the other boy first denied committing the act, but later admitted it, saying 'Well, Albert does it for others.' "

A school official said of Albert:

"Has developed a cunning, subtle attitude of insubordination. Runs after girls in hallways. Found on floors where he has no right to be. Plays truant. Kissed several girls in school. Hugged a smaller boy in school, exclaiming warmly 'My boy, my boy.' Very smooth-spoken, over-sophisticated—has unwholesome influence over boys and girls in school."

Educational authorities urged his mother, Mrs. H., to take Albert to Bellevue Hospital for psychiatric observation, but she was unwilling. At the first court hearing she produced a certificate from an out-of-town psychiatrist stating that Albert was under his care, receiving injections of testosterone propionate (hormones) in an attempt to cure him of homosexuality. At her request she was allowed to continue these treatments over the summer. It was understood that in the fall the matter would be re-evaluated. In September Mrs. H. appeared at court with Albert; she stated that she had had a "nervous breakdown" during the summer and had to quit her job. She expressed a desire to have Albert observed at Bellevue as "he is continually getting into trouble."

It should be noted that when Albert was 5 Mrs. H. gave some very confidential information to a prekindergarten worker. She disclosed that she eloped with Albert's father, Mr. W., when she was 16 and he 18. At the time Albert was 8 months old she discovered that her husband was syphilitic, and Albert was treated for congenital syphilis at a New York hospital. Because Mr. W. deserted her while Albert was still an infant, she boarded him with a woman named C., from whom he has taken his present name. Then Mrs. H. placed him in an orphanage for a year, after which she took him to live with her in her parents' home. She has been keeping company with several men who are critical of Albert. There were suggestions that Mrs. H. engaged intermittently in prostitution.

Albert was remanded to Bellevue Hospital Psychiatric Division in the adolescent ward for boys. He was found to be in good physical condition and of high normal intelligence, but perpetually in conflict with people. He made homosexual advances to other boys, had no feelings of guilt over his activities, and resisted efforts to help him. As he became more at ease with the psychiatrists, he divulged that he has been in one trouble after another ever since he could remember and he did not contemplate any change in behavior. He felt convinced that he could do as he pleased and no one could stop him. A diagnosis was made of psychopathic personality and homosexuality with no evidence of any psychosis at present. It was recommended to the court that Albert be placed on probation and referred to a mental hygiene clinic, but that if there was no improvement in his conduct, he should be placed in an institution.

The court then placed Albert on probation and made arrangements for him to be seen in an excellent mental hygiene clinic, but to no avail. He failed to attend either school or clinic and when placement in a private rehabilitative group was unavailable because his prognosis is very poor, he was committed to a state correctional institution.

It is likely that with his long-established patterns of misconduct Albert will graduate from one offense to other more serious ones, and from Children's Court to adult criminal courts. An inference may be drawn that his mother's continued irregular behavior since before his birth has been a powerful factor contributing to Albert's difficulties.

PETER T.

Peter, who is 14 and in the 7A grade, has been known to a guidance clinic of the Board of Education at intervals for the past four years, having been referred by teachers who described him as insolent, defiant, and disinterested in his subjects. During these periods it was not possible to develop a sustained contact with Peter, who is the younger of two brothers living with their mother. Mr. and Mrs. T. separated when Peter was an infant, and from that time she has been working as a nursing attendant at various hospitals. She expressed deep negative feelings toward her husband, whom she speaks of as an alcoholic and abusive. Since serving a one-year jail sentence for impairing the morals of a minor, his whereabouts have been unknown to his family. Mrs. T. is intelligent, interested in her work, and proud of her good work record. She is especially critical of Peter when his behavior causes her to lose time from work.

Peter's mother told the clinic that he has been nervous from babyhood, sleeps poorly, has nightmares, and sometimes walks in his sleep. He fights, truants, steals, and has remained away from home all night. He is definitely interested in his gang, and she worries about this, fearful that he will become involved in serious trouble with other members. In the clinical psychiatric observation Peter appeared neurotic, overanxious, and exhibited much hostility toward his older brother, who is well behaved and has regular employment. Peter was found to be in need of routine and remedial instruction, but his frequent truancies prevented this. The clinic recommended placement; Mrs. T. was inclined to accept the recommendation as she recognized that he was beyond her control.

When Peter was referred to the court for chronic truancy, the judge remanded him to Bellevue Hospital Psychiatric Division for a three weeks' period of observation. In speaking with the doctors Mrs. T. mentioned that Peter has been a source of trouble since infancy. Ever since he began school he has been quarrelsome and annoying to other children, and she has had constant complaints about him from the school authorities and neighbors. He has had several head injuries and occasionally has dizzy spells. Peter was found to have enlarged, diseased tonsils. A tonsillectomy was advised, but Mrs. T. refused permission for its performance. During the neurological examination an x-ray of the skull was taken which proved negative. Because of Peter's history of head injuries, an electro-encephalogram was done, and it was similar to that seen in patients suffering from convulsive disorders.

On psychometric tests Peter scored an I.Q. of 96 with pronounced retardation in reading and arithmetic. He was able to do only first-grade reading and second-grade arithmetic. His educational retardation has been a severe handicap for him in school. In psychiatric observation Peter was seen to be restless, obscene, quarrelsome, and defiant, and was involved in homosexual practices with a mentally defective boy. He recalled that he has been having sex relations with girls since he was five years old and has been truanting for years. Peter admitted belonging to a gang whose members carry guns and knives, and he himself shot a member of a rival gang with an improvised gun. He has also taken part in thefts and has a very vivid fantasy life in which he is an all-powerful person. The examiners concluded that Peter is an individual of psychopathic personality who may later develop convulsive disorders. At present he is neither psychotic nor mentally deficient, but is suitable for commitment to a correctional institution.

After receiving these findings and recommendation, the judge committed Peter to a state training school for boys. His mother seemed relieved at his departure, for she had feared that before being sent away he would commit a horrible crime. Reports received from the correctional institution indicate that Peter is making a poor adjustment there.

Prognosis is highly unfavorable as Peter's antisocial patterns are well developed, and he is not receptive to the present methods of treatment available in the particular institution.

MARTIN F.

Martin, 13, is the youngest of four children who were born before their parents married. His mother had a child by a previous union whom she "gave" to a relative. After prolonged and intense marital friction over religion, Mr. F. returned to Puerto Rico, where he obtained a divorce from Mrs. F. He is reported to be abusive and cruel, and to have lived on charity and by thefts since he was 8 years old. From the time of his departure two years ago, the family has been receiving public assistance. When Martin was 3, and again when he was 6, he and his siblings lived in foster homes while their mother was hospitalized for tuberculosis. She admits her inability to cope with her children and realizes they need placement until they are old enough to care for themselves.

All of the agencies that have attempted to work with the family concurred in recommending that the children should be placed.

Martin, who has been in classes for pupils with retarded mental development almost from the time he first entered school, was referred to the court for truancy, petty thefts, and bullying younger students. Upon examination at the Bellevue Hospital Mental Hygiene Clinic, he was found to be in good physical condition with borderline intelligence. His I.Q. is 79. When strong antisocial tendencies were observed by the psychiatrist, he made a diagnosis of psychopathic personality and noted that there was no evidence of any psychosis at present. He joined in recommending placement, feeling that unless Martin were protected from himself and society from him grave consequences would follow, because coupled with Martin's definite antisocial patterns were his oversuggestibility and lack of judgment.

Unfortunately, no placement was made at the time because of a feeling that the limited facilities existing should be used for boys who had already committed serious offenses. Several months later Martin was arrested with two other boys for burglarizing a small store, during which the proprietor was shot. They were brought into another branch of the court and are awaiting adjudication.

Prognosis for Martin appears unfavorable, since his antisocial tendencies are already definite and he is likely to be placed in a correctional institution where he will associate with older delinquents who will influence him adversely. His borderline intelligence would mitigate against successful psychotherapy for him even if such treatment were available.

EDWIN O.

Edwin, 14 and a pupil in 6A grade, has a brother, 19, who is serving a prison sentence for robbery, and an older sister who is an inmate of a state school for the feeble-minded. Mr. O. has lived by his wits since the time he was a small boy; he has engaged in petty confidence games and frauds and has exercised more ingenuity and time on these than he would have had to expend in a job. He is said to have told his family that it is silly to work when a person can live on the labor of others. Several times he has spent short periods in jail, but his few court convictions have not dampened his enjoyment of "putting it over on suckers." His parents had died when he was an infant and he had been shunted from one relative to another, none of whom wanted to assume any responsibility for his care.

Mrs. O. was very dull and seemed unable to cope with either her husband or her children. Obese, slow-moving, and bedraggled, she spent most of her time sitting in the kitchen nodding and munching. Two of her sisters had been committed to a state institution for mental defectives, and her father had died of paresis while a patient in a state hospital for the mentally ill. She had never known her mother, who had deserted the family shortly after Mrs. O.'s birth. While working as a waitress in a cheap restaurant, she had met and married Mr. O., dazzled by his free spending and seemingly inexhaustible supply of money and trinkets.

Edwin's parents were indifferent to his nonattendance at school and petty thievery. His mother knew he left the house right after breakfast, but what he did after that seemed of little concern to her if he did not bother her for meals or clothes. Mr. O. thought it was smart of Edwin to fool the teachers by running out of school as soon as roll call was completed and to force younger children to give up their pocket money. When truant officers visited the home, Mr. O. laughed at them and said they were wasting their time, while Mrs. O. sat silently, listened to what they had to say, and closed the door after them. Notes from the school requesting the parents' presence remained unanswered.

Meanwhile, Edwin's truancy and misconduct continued unabated. He became bolder and did not hesitate to use sticks and brass knuckles on children who refused his demands for money and sweets. In class he destroyed their handiwork, shouted whenever others recited, and in the hallways and lavatories made homosexual advances to younger children. They complained to their parents and teachers who, in turn, complained to the school principal. Through his efforts a court referral was made.

When brought to the court, Edwin swaggered and posed. He denied any blame, stating that the others always harassed him instead of recognizing that he was better than they and paying him for playing with them and protecting them from bigger boys. They should have been glad to treat him instead of running to the teachers tattling on him. When asked about his activities, he became sullen and unresponsive. It was recognized that he needed a period of observation in a psychiatric setting, but since no bed would be available for weeks, except for emergency cases, he was remanded to a temporary place of detention until he could be hospitalized.

At the shelter he proved unmanageable, expressing his aggressiveness in assaults upon younger boys, stealing their possessions, destroying these when possible and tormenting them as soon as adults were not present. He cringed before the older boys and sought their favor in various ways. Trying to escape by means of the fire escape, he threw a heavy iron bar at a boy who saw him and barely escaped a fractured skull by darting back. Thereupon the detention authorities asked Bellevue Hospital Psychiatric Division to receive Edwin as an emergency case. They did so and placed him in their adolescent ward.

Medical examination disclosed that Edwin was well developed and well nourished, with many dental caries and impaired vision. Skull x-rays were negative but his electro-encephalograph pattern showed deviations from the norm suggestive of a psychopathic personality. The Rorschach test and psychiatric study in the ward and in interviews confirmed this. He engaged in homosexual activities, fought constantly with younger boys, bullied and threatened them, felt himself at odds with the world, accepted no blame for any of his misdeeds and acknowledged that he has "warred" on others from early childhood. He expressed no intention or desire to change his antisocial habits, feeling it was only natural that he should do his best to torment others and force them to serve him. On psychometric tests he achieved a high average I.Q. of 110, with scholastic retardation in reading and arithmetic. His verbal scores were higher than his performance ones.

After a careful evaluation of their findings, the examining psychiatrists advised that Edwin be committed to a correctional institution, for they believed his chances of an adequate adjustment in the community were very poor, since his antisocial patterns were well developed. Their recommendation was accepted by the court. A report from the state correctional institution to which he was sent indicates that his adjustment there is unsatisfactory.

In view of his family background and psychopathic personality, it is likely that Edwin will continue to transgress. He needs protection from himself and the community needs to be protected from him. Since present science cannot help him sufficiently for him not to be a menace, the state should continue to segregate him and others like him. In that way many violent and horrible crimes could be prevented. Under present legislation and practice, these psychopathic youths are released after a few years to continue their delinquent and criminal careers even though it is known that their destructive patterns of behavior will persist to the detriment of themselves and society.

The Mentally Ill

Occasionally it happens that, unknown to his parents or teachers, a truant is mentally ill. Frequently his ailment is reflected in misbehavior that is a trial to parents and school authorities alike, who become disheartened at his repeated failure to conform with established rules and routines. Naturally, in many of these instances a parent is aware that something is radically amiss but is unable or unwilling to realize the possibility of mental disease and strenuously resists efforts at specific diagnosis and treatment, especially where hospitalization is required. There is almost a belief that reiterated denials of its existence will eliminate the condition.

All the customary fears and feelings of guilt and shame regarding insanity in a family member are intensified and strengthened where one's child is the patient. Yet the most hopeful part and one which many parents can be helped to accept is that the earlier an accurate diagnosis can be made and expert care obtained, the greater are the chances of cure, except of course in most of the organic brain disorders which, fortunately, are rare among young children.

Here, as elsewhere, most parents sincerely wish to do the very best possible for their children. Hence it is fully as much the court's function to aid a parent in accepting his child's illness and secure the parent's active cooperation in planning for diagnosis and treatment as it is to ascertain the basic causes of the child's misconduct and to see that essential specialized services are made available for him. Judges and court workers sometimes find it fully as hard to understand a parent's truculence and vehement protests that "there is nothing wrong with my child" as it is for the same parent to acknowledge the need for expert treatment away from home.

Complications arise where the parent himself is so emotionally disturbed that he is unable to place his child's problem above his own and seems compelled to persist in a damaging and destructive course. The very parental attitudes and behavior that have helped to precipitate the child's mental disorder seem to reach a peak during judicial hearings which stir up latent fears of losing the child. At times the parent is even more seriously ill mentally than his child who has been charged with an offense, and in these cases the court has to proceed authoritatively in the best interests of the child. By recent amendment to the law governing the Children's Court of New York City, its judge may also remand a parent to a psychiatric hospital for observation.[6] Yet unless the adult is in a state of violent mania, he is usually able to negate the remand by the intervention of a relative willing to act as custodian, thus relieving an overcrowded hospital, or by judicial writ freeing him from the institution.

To assist students in understanding the implications involved in the cases that follow, a brief résumé is offered of the major types of mental illnesses affecting children.[7]

[6] Domestic Relations Court Act of the City of New York, Section 61, sub. 7.
[7] Lawson Lowrey, *Psychiatry for Social Workers*. New York, Columbia University Press, 1946. Eugen Blueler, *Textbook of Psychiatry*, trans. by A. A. Brill. New York, Macmillan Co., 1924. Albert Deutsch, *The Mentally Ill in America*. New York, Doubleday-Doran, 1937. Richard H. Hutchings, *A Psychiatric Ward Book*. Utica, N. Y., State Hospitals Press, 1943. Ely Jelliffe and William A. White, *Nervous and Mental Diseases*. Philadelphia, Lee and Febiger, 1915. Karl Menninger, *The Human Mind*. New York, Knopf, 1945.

Dementia praecox, or schizophrenia as it is sometimes termed, and manic-depressive psychosis are the two principal functional mental diseases that are found among children. In the realm of the organic, various forms of brain disorders may exist in young persons. A lesion or atrophy in the central nervous system may be due to accident or other injury, or to unknown causes. Cure is possible for many of those suffering from functional mental disorders, but in our present state of knowledge there is no cure for organic brain disease. Where the brain itself is malformed or damaged, the disorder becomes progressively worse as deterioration advances.

A psychosis usually denotes a deep, far-reaching and prolonged mental disorder characterized by specific symptoms, some of which apply to more than one form of mental disease. Depression and persistent moodiness in an individual may be a symptom of dementia praecox or manic-depressive psychosis, depending upon the other symptoms present. Dementia praecox is a cleavage or disorientation of the mental functions, popularly known as split personality, in which there is substantial withdrawal from reality. The more complete this withdrawal, the more serious is the patient's condition and the less the possibility of recovery. It is said of the schizophrenic that he lives in a dream world, a world of his own. When dementia praecox appears among adolescents, it is connected ordinarily with the outset of puberty and is called hebephrenic type. Delusions of persecution or of grandeur and hallucinations, both auditory and visionary, are other symptoms of schizophrenia. The schizoid must be distinguished from the schizophrenic for the former is not mentally ill but his personality resembles that of the dementia praecox sufferer, as it is shut in, unsocial and introspective, but not to the same degree. However, if the schizoid's condition remains untreated, it may develop into schizophrenia.

A manic-depressive, as the name suggests, is one whose moods vary from extreme, uncontrollable excitement to the depths of despair and misery. These alternate periods of manic excitement and melancholia are also called cyclic insanity, and in some patients the manic stages are dangerously violent, with the melancholia accompanied by strong suicidal impulses.

Where the social worker suspects that a child may be mentally ill, a Rorschach test is valuable, for it can be included in a psychological examination within a guidance unit; in New York City and elsewhere a judicial order is not required for the child's psychological study and destructive delay can be prevented. If the Rorschach pattern is suggestive of a mental disorder, detailed psychiatric and neurological examination should be requested. Particularly in organic brain disease, the electro-encephalograph, skull x-rays, and other neurological procedures have considerable diagnostic value. A period of hospital observation and examination is imperative for full and accurate diagnosis of mental illnesses. Clinical study in an outpatient center is insufficient, although helpful in particular instances as a prelude to hospital study in which the child can be observed on a twenty-four hour a day basis.

It is in relation to securing needed psychiatric hospitalization for a child that the court's remand power is especially valuable. Voluntary admission by parents usually proves ineffectual, for they are prone to have a change of heart even when they know that hospital care is needed, and they proceed to remove him before a complete diagnosis can be made. There are instances in which a parent has removed his child a day or two after admission. Moreover, it is unsound to persuade or force a parent to make such a choice, for natural feelings of guilt are operative and the child, together with other members of the immediate family and relatives, blames the parent for effecting a voluntary commitment. Almost invariably, his change of mind and removal of his child are occasioned by feelings of guilt and the pleas of relatives. The court is in a much better position to arrange for hospitalization and can more easily bear the onus of natural dissatisfactions. Each remand should be timely and sound, predicated upon a foundation of adequate data and skill in evaluating it.

Schizophrenia, Dementia Praecox

Mareo T.

When Mareo was brought into court on a charge of habitual truancy he was 14 and enrolled in the 8A grade. Up to the time of his father's sudden death from heart disease three years previously, Mareo had had an excellent school record both in attendance and scholarship. Since then his record has deteriorated steadily until his absences greatly exceed his attendance. Mareo is an only child who had been strongly attached to his father, a quiet, undemonstrative individual, and felt his loss keenly. Mrs. T., shy, retiring and intelligent, has been receiving public assistance for herself and Mareo from the time of her husband's death. Before that they had managed nicely on his earnings as a mechanic. When asked if she had been having any difficult with Mareo, she told the court that she was deeply worried about him as he had attempted suicide recently by turning on the gas after sealing all the doors and windows. At the time she had gone marketing but found she had forgotten her purse and returned unexpectedly early to find him lying unconscious in their kitchen. Upon reviving him she had inquired why he had tried to take his life; he replied that he was tired of living. Ever since his father's death he has been extremely nervous with severe temper tantrums and bizarre food habits. Lately he has taken to sitting by himself all day in his bedroom, brooding and dreaming.

In view of these circumstances, the court immediately remanded Mareo to Bellevue Hospital for observation and possible commitment to a state institution for the mentally ill. Mrs. T. consented to the remand when she was informed that it was essential to his welfare and that he stood a better chance of recovery if he received treatment at once. On physical examination, Mareo was found to be undernourished, with a lateral curvature of the spine.

Neurological tests were negative, but psychiatric observations disclosed that he was suffering from a severe mental illness—schizophrenia. He had flat emotional tone; low, rambling, and incoherent speech, described auditory hallucinations of long standing, and had such violent emotional outbursts, during which he attacked several other patients, that he had to be transferred from the adolescent ward to a semidisturbed ward. He admitted having attempted suicide, adding that several times since then he has had almost uncontrollable impulses to kill himself. No history of mental disease was indicated for other members of his family.

In psychometric tests Mareo classified as of high average intelligence with an I.Q. of 110 on the Bellevue scale. The test pattern suggested schizophrenia with partial mental deterioration.

After Bellevue Hospital psychiatrists found that Mareo needed care in a state mental hospital, they applied for his commitment to a branch of the Supreme Court located within that hospital. A hearing was held, commitment was ordered, and he was transferred to a state institution for the mentally ill. There he responded well to a program of intensive psychotherapy. He made a fine adjustment, mingling freely with other patients, having a friendly attitude. Almost immediately after admission he requested employment, was assigned to work in the kitchen, and performed his duties rather capably. There was steady improvement physically and mentally with no violent behavior and no relapses.

His mother's request for his release was granted at the end of three months on a convalescent status with the diagnosis of dementia praecox, hebephrenic type (connected with puberty), improved condition and a guarded prognosis. Under the terms of his parole from the hospital, Mareo is obliged to report monthly for treatment in an outpatient center of the State Department of Mental Hygiene. Should he fail to attend or should his condition become worse within a year, he can be brought back to the hospital without court action. If not returned within a year, he is eligible for discharge. Mareo has been readmitted to school and is continuing to receive psychiatric treatment.

It seems almost incredible that in a three-month period Mareo's deep-seated psychosis could have improved so remarkably that outpatient care will be sufficient to prevent relapses. The fact that his mental illness is so intimately connected with puberty may partially account for this, since puberty passes. However, one cannot help but wonder if the hospital's overcrowded condition was not a potent factor in Mareo's quick release, and whether if he had remained there receiving daily help for another three or four months there would be less danger of relapse and more probability of permanent improvement in his condition.

One is also faced with the query: Why was not attention paid to Mareo's behavior before he developed a definite psychosis? If the social workers visiting the home in connection with the grant of public assistance or his teachers had realized the significance of his deteriorating behavior immediately after his father's death, could Mareo's psychosis perhaps have been prevented? Surely it is tragic that nothing constructive was done to help him until fully three years after his behavior deviations were overtly expressed. The importance of early scrutiny and diagnosis of conduct disturbances can hardly be overemphasized.

LEONARD L.

Leonard, 8 years old and a pupil in the 1A grade, is the only child of Mr. L., 28, and Mrs. L., 25, who have been separated ever since his birth. The father, a highly skilled garment worker earning $4,500 annually, cannot bring himself to the point of returning to his wife even for Leonard's sake, because her disorderly habits are unbearable. Mr. L. is devoted to his son and has been saddened at the way in which he has been living with his mother, who persists in treating him as a baby, keeping him out of school the whole semester, and clinging to him day and night. Realizing that Leonard was suffering in this process, his father has besought Mrs. L. to give him custody of the boy, but she has refused. Reluctant to force matters by commencing legal action, Mr. L. has hoped that she would sue him for support in Family Court, at which time he could raise the issue of Leonard's care. But she has preferred not to seek support from him, contenting herself with receiving money from her parents.

When truant officers visited the home they found it to be a shambles of filth, litter, and broken furniture, with Mrs. L. screaming imprecations and insults. They were unable to convince her of the necessity for Leonard's attendance at school. She shouted that neither he nor she liked to see people; they remained at home all day, and whenever she took him to class she noticed he could not do what the other children did. Teachers were aware that he was out of touch with his classmates, was greatly retarded in habit training, and fearful. A referral to court was made on the ground of truancy. Mrs. L. did not respond to summonses and a bench warrant was therefore issued for her and Leonard so that protective action could be taken for him.

Brought into the court by warrant officers who had first tried to persuade her to appear voluntarily, Mrs. L. shouted profanity and threats, leaning all the while on a dirt-padded crutch. Upon inquiry she gave a rambling account of having broken her leg a short time previously but later said this had happened several years ago and that she was perfectly able to walk but liked using a crutch: "It makes me feel good." When asked about Leonard, a small scared boy who clung closely to her and looked like a 5 year old child, she replied that she felt like a child herself and indicated an almost pathological dependence upon her mother. Mrs. L. spoke of Leonard as her infant, her baby from whom she could not bear to be separated long enough for him to attend school.

When she saw Mr. L. in the courtroom, Mrs. L. loudly accused him of conspiring against her and causing her and Leonard to be brought there. Her husband told the court that he has been very anxious about Leonard's "nervousness" and that their family physician had told him Mrs. L.'s emotional imbalance was having an adverse effect upon the child. Mr. L. added that he believed his wife's condition was becoming worse, but she had refused his suggestions of obtaining medical care, nor could her parents prevail upon her to do so. Both her father, a frail, elderly carpenter suffering from an asthmatic heart condition, and her mother, a quiet, gentle, hard-working woman, were distressed and disturbed by her outbursts.

After a remand had been ordered for her and Leonard to be observed at Bellevue Hospital Psychiatric Division, Mrs. L. became hysterical and threatened to beat the attendants and the judge with her crutch. She could not be persuaded to go quietly and had to be removed bodily. The examining psychiatrists found her to be suffering from schizophrenia and recommended that she be committed to a state hospital. However, her mother interceded, pleading to be allowed to have custody of Mrs. L. and promising that she would no longer interfere in Leonard's development. Thereupon she was released on the condition that she relinquish Leonard until she was mentally fit to have him.

Hospital authorities made a full study of Leonard. Physically he was in good condition except for a severe strabismus of the eyes (squint) with a visual defect. Neurological examination showed the primitive reflex responses which are characteristic of both retarded and schizophrenic children. The electro-encephalogram revealed generalized dysthymia (functional disorder) found in problem children. On psychometric tests Leonard scored an I.Q. of 72, borderline intelligence, although it was felt that his innate ability was much higher. Due to psychotic factors and scholastic retardation, he was functioning at a borderline level with poorly developed social concepts. Psychiatric observations revealed that Leonard was suffering from childhood schizophrenia or dementia praecox. He was intensely preoccupied, had to be carefully supervised as to feeding, toilet, and sleeping habits, clung to another child, ran around in a restless, aimless fashion, had many strong fantasies, and an ambivalent (shifting) attitude toward his mother. His serious mental ailment was attributed in large measure to his mother's disordered behavior. It was recommended that he be remanded back to the hospital for a month's psychotherapy.

The court followed the recommendation, and at the end of the period Leonard's condition had improved so markedly that additional shock therapy was recommended to be done either in a clinic or by a private psychiatrist. It was emphasized that he should not be permitted to live with his mother for some time to come as this would cause serious relapse. Mr. L. arranged for Leonard to attend a private boarding school and receive private psychiatric treatment. At the end of six months it was almost impossible to recognize him as the same boy who had been brought into court before. He was alert, well oriented, and had lost his expression of fear and trepidation. Reports from school and psychiatrist indicated that his progress was satisfactory, and he was therefore discharged from the court's supervision and with an order confirming the award of Leonard's custody to his father.

Despite his mother's patently destructive influences, it was possible to help Leonard because he received timely hospitalization and expert treatment. It is too bad that no court referral was made until after his mental disorder had developed into a psychosis, as both he and his father could have been spared much suffering. Immediately upon Leonard's reaching the compulsory school age of 7, the reasons for his absences could have been determined and action begun. Nevertheless, the school authorities deserve credit for commencing court action before he passed into successive grades with his basic problems untouched. It is not to be wondered at that his father did not initiate court action as he had had a long series of painful experiences with his wife and hesitated to precipitate others.

A negative factor that ought not be overlooked is Mrs. L.'s continued presence in the community untreated and thus becoming more seriously ill as time goes on. Her elderly parents cannot cope with her successfully and as soon as her fright over her observation period subsides, her need for Leonard will rise to the fore and she will seek him and try her best to have him restored to her. Whether or not her husband will be able to garner sufficient strength to prevent this is problematical. It is likely that if she attempts to do so within the next few years, he will seek the aid of the court which awarded him custody, although the combined pleas of Leonard and Mrs. L. may cause Mr. L. to weaken.

GILBERT H.

Gilbert, 14 and a pupil in the 6A grade, was referred to the Bureau of Child Guidance by school authorities, who noticed that he sat in the classroom grinning constantly, breaking out into mad laughter, unable to do any assignments, and hiding in clothes closets. Their psychologist was unable to determine Gilbert's intellectual status because of his serious emotional disturbance. Social service exchange reports disclosed that Gilbert and his parents had been known to several private agencies, including the National Desertion Bureau. After prolonged marital friction culminating in repeated desertions, Mr. and Mrs. H. were divorced and she was awarded Gilbert's custody. In a contact two years previously, a social worker had noted that Gilbert was unable to play with boys in the neighborhood; his mother was not able to handle him adequately; he seemed very insecure in his relationship to her, demanded a great deal of attention and continually clung to her. Another agency obtained more background material from Mrs. H., who was guarded and protective in talking with their worker. She had requested them a year and a half earlier to place him in camp for the summer, but it was apparent that he was very disturbed and not suitable for a camp placement. Her manner was rigid and hostile, revealing little warmth for Gilbert; her exasperation and complete sense of failure were evident.

Mrs. H. described her early home as happy and comfortable, although her father was domineering and she still feared him. Her husband had a master's degree from a well-known college, but was unemployed when she married him at 20 and has never held a steady job, occasionally having a clerical job which he would work at for several months and then quit. He considered most work beneath him, did not provide a home for her, and, after intense quarrels, left her four times before their final separation, which occurred at the time of Gilbert's birth. Before her marriage she had completed high school and had good musical training but went into factory work. Neither parent wanted a child and Mrs. H. was tearful and upset throughout her pregnancy. She worked until Gilbert was born prematurely. Then she spent all her savings for his care in an incubator for two months. Mr. H. told her to name the baby "Unwelcome" and she had felt like doing so.

Living with her parents and working during Gilbert's earliest years, Mrs. H. had little time for Gilbert, who has been a feeding problem since infancy. She and her parents always felt they had to entertain him in order to get him to eat. He became almost unmanageable when he started school. Neither his grandparents nor his mother could cope with him, and he did about as he pleased with few exceptions. His aggressiveness seemed to be a defense against fear and timidity. He expressed fear that the social worker would take him away, as his grandmother had often threatened him with placement. When he was 6 he had been sent to camp, where he refused to eat or sleep. At home his mother always shared a room with him, and if she did not retire with him he refused to go to bed. Her attitude toward him seemed one of deep-seated rejection, and his grandmother seemed equally incapable of setting up any controls for him. The grandfather had tried to discipline Gilbert, but neither his wife nor Mrs. H. would permit him to do so. Mr. H. had not seen Gilbert in more than four years and evinced no interest in him.

Under these circumstances the agency tried to help Mrs. H. place Gilbert, but she was opposed to placement.

Approximately a year later Mrs. H. was induced by her parents to have Gilbert examined in a mental hygiene clinic because he refused to leave the house, was seclusive, sat in class without showing any interest in his subjects. According to his mother Gilbert "was becoming childish. He acts foolish and laughs all the time for no reason." No adequate measure of his intelligence was possible because of his extreme disturbance. Medical examinations showed him to be in good physical condition except for obesity. In psychiatric interviews he had a perpetual grin, was unresponsive, evasive, withdrawn, defensive, immature, childish, simple, apathetic, and emotionally flat. His general behavior, responses and reactions were those of a schizophrenic boy, and the diagnosis made was schizophrenia. The psychiatrist recommended to Mrs. H. that she take Gilbert to Bellevue Hospital Psychiatric Division, but she refused to do so.

When the Bureau of Child Guidance received these reports, Mrs. H. was asked to come in for discussion. After she failed to keep two appointments, the principal was advised to suspend Gilbert and request an administrative hearing before an assistant superintendent. A representative of the Bureau was present at the hearing and was impressed by Mrs. H.'s emotional instability and defensiveness. She agreed to place Gilbert at Bellevue Hospital for observation, but when it was learned that she had not taken him there after arrangements had been made, the child was brought into court so that necessary psychiatric care could be obtained for him.

At the court hearing, despite Mrs. H.'s hysterical opposition, Gilbert was remanded to Bellevue Hospital Psychiatric Division for observation and possible commitment to a state hospital for the mentally ill. She was impervious to any attempt at explanation, and her behavior was indicative of a disintegrating personality. Her attitudes and conduct during several hospital visits to Gilbert led the psychiatrists to conclude that she would soon need hospitalization in an institution for mental diseases. Gilbert was found to be in good physical condition except for obesity, with an increased distribution of fat about the hips and in the breast regions. On the Bellevue intelligence scale he achieved an I.Q. of 43, but this score was not considered representative of his native endowment because the test pattern showed many signs of schizophrenia.

Psychiatric examination revealed a bizarre appearing boy with a constant vacuous smile who avoided all contact with other patients and ward personnel. He never joined a group even at mealtimes, preferring to eat by himself. During interviews he was preoccupied, nonspontaneous, rambling, and incoherent. His thinking processes were distorted and he used vague notions instead of concrete representations. Gilbert had lost affective contact with his environment, and it was impossible to establish any rapport with him. His outward emotional display was always inappropriate, never in harmony with the thought content. Vague auditory and visual hallucinations of an indefinite nature were elicited. His judgment was markedly impaired and he lacked insight.

These findings led to a diagnosis of schizophrenia, hebephrenic type. In all probability this condition has existed for some time, becoming progressively worse. The examining psychiatrists therefore applied for Gilbert's admission to the children's ward of a state hospital for the mentally ill. He was admitted upon an order of commitment and immediately began receiving psychotherapy. Their report suggests that the prognosis for Gilbert is poor, primarily because treatment has been so long delayed.

Gilbert's mental illness is seen to be even more serious than Mareo's, despite the fact that Mareo's behavior was the more violent of the two, for Gilbert's retreat from reality is more complete and of longer standing. It may be due to the destructive influences of his parents, practically from the time of his conception, aggravated by his mother's steadily deteriorating behavior, the onset of puberty and the lack of timely treatment. From the time he first entered school there existed evidence of his increasingly severe mental disturbance. Why did it take until he reached 14 before a court referral was made? Here is illustrated the concept that overt misbehavior annoying to teachers in its manifestations, such as fighting, insolence and defiance is more apt to be noticed and acted upon than extreme quietness and seclusion which are symptomatic of more serious emotional disturbances. Teachers need to be as alert in noticing those indications that usually do not present discipline problems as those that do. When a number of Gilbert's teachers were queried by the court, most of them responded that they had given him fair marks and had passed him along from one grade to another because he wasn't "bad" or noisy, did not fight, and tried even though he could not do class assignments. Only his current teacher, who had suggested the referral to the Bureau of Child Guidance, realized that Gilbert's dreaminess and extreme quietness were indicative of something amiss and informed the principal that it was impossible to grade Gilbert in any of his subjects. If only such a referral had been made before Gilbert's mental disturbance had developed into a psychosis, or even before his psychosis had become so severe, he could have been spared so much unhappiness and disintegration.

In Gilbert's case there is also exemplified the futility of expecting compliance with suggestions for placement of a child from a parent who is so emotionally upset as Mrs. H. Six months' delay in treatment could have been prevented had there been a court referral as soon as the guidance unit recognized the severity of Gilbert's disorder, the disturbance of Mrs. H., and her persistent disapproval of his placement as disclosed in interviews and social service reports.

ARTHUR M.

Arthur, 7, an only child, and in the 2A grade, was suspended from school because of violent outbursts of temper and fights with other children and teachers. Thereupon the Bureau of

Attendance referred him to court as a discipline problem. After incessant and bitter quarrels from the time of their marriage, Mr. and Mrs. M. were divorced when Arthur was 5. His mother then took him to her parents' home where both have continued to reside together with Mrs. M.'s sister, who supports the entire household. Mr. M. remarried almost immediately but has no children by his second wife. He impressed the court as very immature and dull but interested in Arthur. Mr. M.'s antipathy toward his first wife was marked. She also seemed dull and ineffectual, as well as dependent, trying hard to love Arthur, despite her deep aversion to his conduct. She expressed considerable anxiety about his behavior.

Social service exchange reports disclosed significant data. A year previously Arthur had been known to the children's health class of a well-known hospital where he was found to have dull normal intelligence and was felt to be reacting to a difficult home condition. Accordingly, he and his mother had been referred to a private family agency which noted that she was upset and guilty about Arthur's "sickness"—his aggression, nocturnal fears, and food fads, but she appeared unable to follow the agency's treatment suggestions. Several months later, as Arthur's difficulties increased, she admitted an inability to deal with his "wildness" and placed him in a private child-caring institution. After remaining there five months, Arthur was discharged as "completely unable to adapt himself to group living" and Mrs. M. was advised to place him in a foster home, but she was emotionally unable to accept this.

Then he had been readmitted to public school, but his misconduct grew worse and the school referred him to a psychiatric clinic. There he was found to be reacting to an extremely insecure relationship with his mother and a destructive home. The clinic tried to arrange for psychiatric observation of Arthur, but was unable to do so. They described Mrs. M. as a person of limited intelligence and insight, unable to act upon their placement recommendation for Arthur. They considered his father to be a psychopathic personality and found that he and other relatives were continually fighting over Arthur. In psychometric tests given in the clinic, he scored an I.Q. of 74, but this was not regarded as accurately representing his innate ability due to variabilities reflecting emotional upset.

The clinic then called upon a child placement agency to help

Mrs. M. and Arthur. After examining the boy their psychiatrist reported:

"There are several reasons why I question foster home placement for Arthur. First of all, the mother's ambivalence and his enormous demands make it doubtful whether either will accept a foster home. More serious is my concern about the profound degree of disturbance which he manifests. His confusion and the bizarre quality of his productions point to a degree of neurotic conflict which may border on the psychotic. The present indication before placement is for more intensive psychiatric study, preferably in a hospital."

The court referral was then made.

During the first court hearing Mrs. M. acknowledged her inability to handle Arthur and upon inquiry expressed a willingness to accept a remand for him at Bellevue Hospital Psychiatric Division, adding that she was frightened at his attempts to tear his flesh and to choke himself. At the hospital's request he was observed and treated there for a three months' period. He was found to be physically well developed, moderately obese, of dull normal intelligence, and suffering from a state of severe anxiety. The Rorschach test pattern showed a deep, overwhelming anxiety and insecurity. Observations on the ward and in psychiatric interviews confirmed these findings. He had frequent dreams of his home going up in flames, of his parents burning to death, etc. His anxieties were the most severe of any child in the hospital, and he had a definite mental illness—schizophrenia. The psychiatrists informed his mother that they would like to treat him with electric shock and she gave her permission. Although he showed some improvement under this therapy, it was not altogether satisfactory.

After their thorough study, the hospital recommended to the court that Arthur should be placed in a child-caring institution with normal children. It has been their experience that schizophrenic children sometimes show improvement after shock treatment when they have been placed in a normal environment. Despite every effort to make such a placement, the court was unable to do so, since there existed no such public facilities and the private institutions having vacancies were unwilling to admit Arthur in view of his mental illness. They felt his presence would be prejudicial to the other children residing there. The court had no alternative except to parole Arthur in his mother's custody, although the hospital had advised against this.

Two months later Arthur became exceedingly upset and tried to leap out of a fourth story window in his home. Mrs. M. called an ambulance which returned him to Bellevue Hospital Psychiatric Division. Another period of observation confirmed their previous opinion that Arthur has childhood schizophrenia and has not benefited much from treatment. With his mother's consent he was therefore transferred to the children's ward of a state hospital for the mentally ill, with a poor prognosis.

One can understand readily the position of the private child-caring groups who felt it inadvisable to accept Arthur. Their programs are geared to the needs of normal children whose welfare they are obliged to place above the needs of a single child such as Arthur, who undoubtedly would benefit more from association with mentally well boys and girls than with other mentally ill children. It is a case of the welfare of the group taking precedence over the welfare of an individual. Still, it is hard to conceive that outstanding psychiatrists at Bellevue would have made such a recommendation if they considered that his presence would be in any way inimical to that of others within a group. The community owes a duty to these ill youngsters to provide them with public facilities necessary to their recovery. The time must come when facilities will exist for all child sufferers in a great metropolitan area like New York City.

Another point worth noting here is that in order for the court to help Arthur by making psychiatric treatment available to him, it had to label him a delinquent. Under present legislation the court has jurisdiction over alleged neglected, dependent, and delinquent children and can exercise its powers to help these children only. Arthur could not be termed either a dependent or a neglected child, since he was supported by his family, who were providing the best physical and emotional care for him within the limits of their capacities. That left the label of delinquent, which technically was applicable in view of his school misconduct, which resulted in expulsion. Yet to call a 7 year old child delinquent because his mental illness is manifested in disturbed behavior is ironic. The legislation in question should be amended so as to enable the court to assist such children without the taking of a delinquency petition.

Manic-Depressive Psychosis

Ruth S.

Ruth, 15 and a student in the second year of high school, was referred to the court for habitual truancy. She is the youngest of three girls whose father deserted their home five years previously after repeated violent quarrels, and whose mother, an intelligent, excitable, hard-working woman, supported them in part by sewing. From before Ruth's birth the family has been aided by relief agencies, first private and then public, for even while he was with them Mr. S. did not work steadily. He has not been heard of by the family since Ruth was 2 years old. Ruth's next oldest sister, Mildred, is the most stable member of the family. Her husband, an accountant is very fond of his wife's family.

When a new public welfare worker first visited the home last year, she noticed that Ruth was overexcited, stubborn, and disobedient. Mrs. S. then told this worker that "no one could do anything with Ruth"; Mrs. S. was considering placing Ruth. The worker then referred them to a guidance agency which found on checking with the school that Ruth had been called to the visiting teacher's attention three years previously for excitability, impertinence, disobedience, and irregularity in attendance. Mrs. S. had mentioned to the teacher that Ruth remained out with boys until 3 A.M., had temper tantrums during which she lay on the floor screaming, and created turmoil in school. However, as her school work was satisfactory and she passed all her subjects and achieved an I.Q. of 104 in a group test, the matter was dropped.

In the guidance unit Ruth gradually established a relationship with her social worker after a period of evasiveness. Ruth verbalized her difficulties somewhat: She felt rejected by her mother in favor of the eldest sister. Consequently, Ruth was lonely, unhappy, jealous, regretful of not being a boy, liking to imitate boys and feeling as though she were not a girl. She felt that there was something wrong with her as she became greatly excited whenever she sang and became so hilarious while at a dance that all the other guests commented upon it. A few days later she felt very sad and as though something in her chest was tearing her to pieces. At such times she did not know what to do with herself. All her life she has had dreadful fears. Very often when she was about 6 years old she liked to go down to the "water's edge" of the East River, try to measure the depth of the water, and see how far she would jump to be submerged. During these times she had a strong wish to drown herself and in order not to do so would run away from the pier. She has continued to have the impulse to drown herself. On many occasions she was positive that men followed her, and she believed that once she kicked one, then crushed him. She "saw" men on rooftops peering in at her and watching her for hours at a time. Ruth also expressed a deep fear of rats, adding that she protected herself by sitting on top of the kitchen table most of the morning. On one occasion she threatened to jump out of a fifth story window, but her mother and sister prevented the leap.

After the staff psychiatrist of the guidance agency had reviewed their case data, he felt that Ruth had presented very disturbed behavior difficulties since her early childhood and that her mental state had taken a decided turn for the worse. He was convinced that her condition was so serious that it could not be treated successfully on an outpatient basis and advised that she should be remanded to Bellevue Hospital Psychiatric Division.

Ruth's extreme excitement alternating with depression was noticeable before and during the court hearing, and it was felt best that she be remanded to Bellevue at once. There she was found to be in good physical condition. Neurological tests, including an electro-encephalogram, were negative. On psychometic examination she scored an I.Q. of 87, placing her functioning at a dull normal level. Her uneven and atypical performance suggested that her score was not truly representative of her native ability. She tended to be hasty, impatient, and negativistic, but when admonished she controlled herself for a time. Little self-criticism was noted, and as soon as tasks were at all hard, she refused to try. She revealed unusually poor comprehension and her functioning throughout the psychological tests raised a question of a psychosis. Her Rorschach pattern was indicative of a psychopathic personality who was so suspicious and distrustful that her thinking and behavior were psychotic.

Psychiatric observation disclosed Ruth to be mentally ill, but her symptoms were so suggestive of both manic-depressive psychosis and paranoia that her psychosis could not be classified at the time and was listed as an undiagnosed psychosis. Emotionally she swung from hilarity and explosive outbursts to periods of depression during which she was suicidal. In addition, she was paranoid to the point where she believed that the teachers, principals, and all students were plotting against her and that she was one of the most popular students and that this was why most of the teachers were against her. On the ward she varied greatly from an overactive, restless but jovial girl to an irritable, hostile patient. The hospital suggested to the family that Ruth be committed to a state institution for the mentally ill, but the mother and sisters were unwilling and instead made arrangements for her to be treated by a private psychiatrist who advised that while under his care she make her home with Mildred. This plan was acceptable to the hospital so the court raised no objection but kept Ruth under supervision for eight months as a protection to her.

Reports received from her psychiatrist indicated that she has quieted down and her delusions of persecution are subsiding. He believes her condition is still serious and will require treatment for approximately a year longer. Mildred and her husband are paying the fees and feel that Ruth is making a satisfactory adjustment in their home.

One wonders why psychiatric treatment was not made available to Ruth long before she reached 15, since her symptoms were evident years ago and the family was known to case work agencies since before her birth. It is tragic that not until her mental state developed into a psychosis was a diagnosis made and care obtained, yet behavior patterns similar to hers are discussed in social work courses.

Possible Brain Disorders

CLIFFORD O.

Clifford, 15½ and in the first term of high school was brought into court on a charge of chronic truancy. Before his case was heard he ran out of the building, but he was apprehended on a warrant and remanded to a temporary shelter for full study. While there he tried to kill another boy with a knife and threw a piece of iron out of a window, which barely missed a young woman who was passing by. The shelter authorities felt he was beyond their control and requested his transfer. The court therefore remanded Clifford to Bellevue Hospital Psychiatric Division for a three weeks' observation period.

Clifford is large for his age and well built. According to his parents, who are separated, he has had no serious illness but has had a head injury due to an automobile accident. He used to live with his father, a barber, who is quiet and law abiding. When Clifford was in trouble at one school for petty thefts and fighting he went to live with his mother in order to obtain a transfer to another school. Mrs. O. works steadily as a seamstress; she appears to be stable and well integrated. Both parents are fearful that Clifford will become involved in serious trouble. They have cooperated with school authorities but are unable to control Clifford, who is a member of a well-organized street gang known to the police for assaults, thefts, and fights with guns and knives. Several times the police have arrested Clifford for participating in these brawls but have released him upon finding that he is under 16. When he was taken to Bellevue he became abusive toward his parents, threatening that he would kill them.

Physical examination showed Clifford to be well developed and well nourished. His electro-encephalogram was abnormal, showing diffuse but no localizable electrocortical dysrhythmia. X-ray of the skull was normal. In psychometric tests Clifford achieved an I.Q. of 88 on the Bellevue scale, classifying as dull normal. The Rorschach pattern suggested a highly disturbed personality, deep insecurity. He experienced great difficulty in establishing or maintaining relationships with other people and displayed negativistic tendencies. Although he refused to cooperate in educational tests, there were indications of substantial retardation in reading and arithmetic.

Upon admission to the hospital he had to be placed in a disturbed ward because of his violence and resistence, screaming that everyone was against him and hated him. When he became quiet he was transferred to a convalescent ward, but adjusted so poorly that he was sent to a semidisturbed ward where he remained for the rest of the remand period. During psychiatric interviews he was sullen, resentful, defensive, and careful not to give any information that he felt might be detrimental to him. He conceded that he was quarrelsome, had temper outbursts and frequent fights, but felt justified and without blame. In his opinion it was perfectly all right to throw the piece of iron out of the window as it was in his way and it would not be his fault if the iron injured a passer-by; that would have been an accident. He had no overt guilt feelings and at times his attitude resembled that of a paranoid. Attempts to help him understand his unstable behavior proved futile.

The examining psychiatrists concluded that Clifford was not psychotic at this time but had a severe personality disorder, partly on a neurotic basis, but also possibly the result of an organic brain disturbance due to a head injury. They felt it unlikely that he would adjust satisfactorily in the community in view of his quarrelsome and assaultive behavior patterns, recognizing that it is hard for him to control his impulsive reactions to the slightest provocations. It was recommended that he be committed to a correctional institution where he would receive adequate supervision. At a court hearing in which the issue of his commitment was raised, both parents pleaded earnestly that he be discharged to either of them so that he might have "another chance." Moved by their pleas, the judge ordered Clifford released to his mother. Several months later he was involved in an assault and robbery but escaped apprehension by disappearing from the state.

Prognosis for Clifford's social adjustment is poor. He probably will proceed from one form of delinquent activity to another, each characterized by aggression and impulsiveness. With time his brain abnormality may become even more serious and be reflected in increasingly violent misconduct.

For his own protection and that of society he should have been committed to a correctional institution in line with the psychiatrists' recommendation.

ROLAND W.

Roland, 14 and enrolled in the 6A grade, is the youngest of three children whose mother is a widow earning their living as a highly skilled domestic. Frank, 17, is an excellent student in a school for mechanical trades, and Agnes, 16, does good work in a commercial high school, attending to household duties in the afternoons. Mr. W., who died of cancer four years previously, had worked steadily as a chauffeur. Among both parents and children there were warm, harmonious relationships. Mrs. W. and her two older children have been increasingly anxious about Roland who has been in one scrape after another for the past two years, culminating in his expulsion from school and subsequent referral to court on charges of habitual truancy and classroom misconduct.

When playing with other children, Roland would become violently assaultive, striking them and destroying their toys. In class he was unduly restless, defiant, disruptive, and belligerent, threatening fellow pupils and teachers. Oftentimes he would leave the building while classes were in session and would disappear for several days while family members searched for him. He liked to carry small sharp knives and would jab these at any child with whom he became angry. During his temper outbursts, which were frequent, he seemed utterly unable to control himself. Failures were recorded in all his school subjects, as he neither tried nor was able to recite or pass tests.

Upon inquiry by the courts, Mrs. W. related that about two and a half years prior to the interview, Roland had suffered a head injury as a result of an automobile accident. He had spent two months in a hospital, then had convalesced at home for another month before returning to school. Ever since then he has had severe headaches and temper tantrums. Before that he was an even tempered and a well behaved boy. She was fearful that he would stab someone and be arrested, but did not know where to seek help for him. She had hesitated to take court action, feeling that he and her other children would blame her for "going to the authorities." She appeared relieved that the court now shared responsibility with her for Roland.

When the advisability of an observation period for him was discussed with her, she did not oppose a remand to Bellevue Hospital Psychiatric Division. There he was found to be physically well developed and well nourished, but neurological tests revealed the existence of an organic brain disease which showed signs of becoming progressively worse. Skull x-rays and electroencephalograms showed organic deviations which were attributed to the head injuries which Roland had received when he was struck by an automobile about two years before. No history of mental disorder was elicited for any other member of his family. Because of his mental condition, psychometric examinations could not be completed and hence no accurate I.Q. could be obtained. His Rorschach pattern was indicative of malfunctioning of the brain. These findings were borne out in psychiatric observations on the ward and in interviews. Roland's uncontrollable aggressive impulses found expression in violent episodes and he had to be transferred to a disturbed ward.

Under these circumstances the psychiatrists advised that Roland be committed to a state hospital for the mentally ill, for if he were permitted to remain in the community he would be a menace to himself and to others. Mrs. W. offered no opposition to this plan as she was convinced of its soundness, and accordingly he was transferred to a state institution.

Prognosis here is poor as in the opinion of experts Roland's brain is deteriorating and there exists no known remedy for his condition.

It is fortunate that Roland was removed from the community before he had committed a serious crime. His mother's realistic attitude aided both the court and the hospital in helping him.

CHAPTER VI

THE PHYSICALLY ILL AND THE SOCIALLY HANDICAPPED

PERUSAL of court records indicates that on occasion serious physical illness may be the primary causal factor producing delinquency. In most of these instances neither the child himself, his family, nor the school knew that he was ill. At times the medical condition was of long standing and becoming progressively worse but was not observed in the hurried routine examinations which overworked school health personnel conducted. Boys whose vision is so defective that they cannot see the blackboard and develop blinding headaches when they try to read their textbooks have, in desperation, remained away from school without realizing the cause of their discomfort. Students with impaired vision or hearing or severe respiratory infections have fled from the demands of class attendance.

A large variety of medical problems is represented, ranging from congenital syphilis, tuberculosis, and glandular imbalance to diabetes, heart disease, and ear defects. Until thorough physical examinations at frequent intervals become an integral part of our educational system in elementary school, junior high, and high schools, this deplorable condition will continue to exist. Medical follow-up work through private family physicians and clinics is a correlative responsibility, since sometimes parents, even when apprised of the matter, are lax in obtaining needed care.

THOMAS F.

Thomas, 12 years old, was referred to the court on a charge of habitual truancy, having absented himself for most of two semesters. His school record up to that time was excellent. Neither his teachers nor his parents could understand the change. When asked why he did not go to school, he shrugged his shoulders and replied that he did not know; he could not stand being indoors. He spent most of his time near the waterfront. Mr. and Mrs. F. were worried about Tom. They were surprised to find that he did not attend classes, for he would leave the house each morning on time, taking his books, carfare, and lunch money. Mr. F., an accountant, was companionable with his three children and felt grief stricken at the thought of one being in court. There had been no difficulty with the other children, nor with Tom at any previous time.

When Tom was interviewed by the court social worker she noted that he kept breathing through his mouth and that his nasal passages seemed blocked. He did not appear to be getting enough air even though the windows were open. She asked Tom about this. He responded that he had not noticed anything wrong except that he always longed to be outdoors and that at night it was hard for him to sleep because his nose and throat would "feel all stuffed up." Immediately full medical examination was arranged for Tom and the report recommended surgery for the removal of a nasal obstruction. His parents were informed and they had the operation performed as quickly as possible. After a short period of convalescence Tom returned to school and has been attending regularly. He told the court worker that he feels so much better and has gained eleven pounds in the past two months. By tutoring in mathematics and grammar, he has made up his work so that he will be promoted at the end of the term with his classmates and feels happy about it.

If the school authorities or his parents had been sufficiently observant here Tom would not have had to be referred to court. His parents were able and willing to cooperate in securing essential medical attention for Tom. This case is typical of many which can and should be settled outside of court.

ROGER T.

Roger, 9 years of age and in 3A grade, was referred to the court for persistent truancy. His mother, a widow with four older children, was in despair because when she brought him to school he would run out of the classroom after roll was taken. She feels he is a bright boy as he learns readily at home and makes fine small airplanes. He plays well with other children and they like him, always seeking him out as a companion. From all accounts the T. family is respectable and hard-working. Mrs. T. has a small income which is supplemented by her two older daughters' earnings. She remains at home, keeping a well-run household for the family.

While interviewing Roger, the court social worker observed that he had trouble hearing her and sometimes failed to respond, not because he did not know the answer, but because he had not heard the question. Upon inquiry he stated that his seat was in the last row of the classroom and that oftentimes he could not hear what his teacher or the other students had said. The worker then scheduled medical and psychological examinations for Roger in the court's clinic. Back came the reports: On the psychometric tests Roger had an I.Q. of 110, intellectually capable of doing fine schoolwork, with some retardation in arithmetic due, in the examiner's opinion, to defective hearing. Physically, Roger is in good shape except for impaired hearing in his right ear, for which an operation was recommended.

These findings were discussed with Roger's mother who was greatly relieved that the problem was not more serious. Responsibility was left with her to carry out the recommendation, which she gladly did. Subsequent reports show that Roger had returned to school, and there is no difficulty about his attendance. He is happy that the truant officer no longer has to come to the house.

It is a pity that Roger's impaired hearing was not discovered and treated without a court referral. It is the school's responsibility to detect such a condition and to seek parental cooperation.

MARTIN C.

Martin is 15 years of age and in 9B grade. His two older brothers are in military service. After years of conflict and nonsupport, Mrs. C. refused to re-establish a home with Mr. C., an engineer whose license was revoked for unethical business practices. She earns a livelihood for Martin and herself by working as a stenographer. There has been no question about Martin's conduct until last semester. Until then his school record was one of steady attendance and progress in all subjects. After he was promoted to a rapid class because of high marks, he asked to be placed in a regular class. He was asked to await the next marking period. Persistent truancy then followed. Shortly thereafter the grade placement he had requested was made, but he did not return to class.

A few months previously Martin had been referred to a hospital by the school doctor for marked obesity and underdevelopment of the genital organs. He was seen in the Children's Endocrine Clinic where intensive endocrine therapy was begun under a diagnosis of adipose genital dystrophy with hypogonadism. Martin came to the clinic for two months, then destroyed the remaining medication and refused to report back for further treatment. Although urged to continue, he refused, with the embarrassment that a sensitive adolescent would have at the examinations and medication essential for his ailment. The marked underdevelopment of his genitals imposed a psychological strain on Martin. It is possible that other boys remarked on his condition.

When Martin was referred to the the court for habitual truancy, a letter of inquiry was sent to the clinic, and in reply it was emphasized that his age and diagnosis make it imperative for him to have consistent and persistent treatment if there is to be any improvement in his condition. Since Martin's cousin, a very reputable physician, offered to give him the necessary treatments in a private office, the court encouraged him to accept this service. After a period of medication Martin returned to school. It is interesting to note that his I.Q. is 128, and once he was back at school he enjoyed his studies.

If the school had had a social worker, it is likely that similar arrangements could have been completed without the necessity for court action.

VAL M.

Val is 13 and in the 6A grade. He is gaunt, undersized, and listless, the middle member of a family with siblings ranging from 2 to 24 years of age. There is a complete lack of parental control in Val's family, as his father is serving in the merchant marine and his mother is bedridden with cancer. Val's two oldest brothers are in the Navy, and his only adult sister is married and lives elsewhere. The apartment is neat with sufficient sleeping quarters for all members of the family, but the neighborhood is in the heart of a delinquency area.

When Val was referred to the court for habitual truancy, a check of his school record showed repeated failures and unexplained school absences since the fourth grade. The court scheduled medical, psychological, and psychiatric examinations for Val, and in these the most significant finding was that he was suffering from tuberculosis and required immediate hospitalization. This was arranged. Other findings were dull normal intelligence with severe educational retardation, especially in reading and arithmetic, but no marked psychiatric deviations.

Here again the school should have ascertained Val's medical problem without referring him to court. He is a physically ill boy, not a delinquent.

The Socially Handicapped

In the following cases careful study discloses that truancy and other misdeeds were caused not by mental or emotional factors but by social factors, principally adverse family conditions. By reacting with truancy and allied habits some of these children were trying to escape from unbearable homes and their reactions were healthful and normal. Even though in some instances improvements were possible while the child remained at home, in the majority placement was the only feasible solution. Unfortunately, even where badly needed, a suitable substitute home was not always available. What these boys and girls required was an opportunity to acquire new habits in a regularized regime with other normal children. Lack of adequate supervision is seen to be a potent force in the development of truancy and other misbehavior. Despite educators' feeling that these children were delinquent, for the most part they were neglected, or they became delinquent primarily because of neglect.

As in other groups, individual study was needed before mental retardation, medical problems, emotional disturbance, or mental illness could be ruled out as causative agents producing misconduct. Examination in an outpatient clinic was usually sufficient, but on occasion a period of hospital observation was essential for accurate diagnosis. Individual study is an imperative prerequisite to effective placement, so that the type of substitute home best suited to the child's own needs may be sought. The most progressive of the private placement agencies and institutions will not consider a child for admission until after their intake committees have received and evaluated social, medical, psychological, and psychiatric data concerning him. By this means they can determine more effectively whether or not he will fit into their program and be benefited by it.

ANTHONY AND ANGELO T.

Anthony, 15½ and enrolled in the second year of a vocational high school, and his brother, Angelo, 14 and a pupil in the 7A grade, have a younger sibling, Charles. Both were referred to the court for persistent truancy. When they were small their parents were divorced after Mr. T. deserted his family. He has continued to reside in another state and has not seen his sons for many years. For approximately five years from the time of their father's desertion, Anthony and Angelo lived in religious institutions, placed there by their mother, a frail, nervous, overanxious woman who was described as a nagger. She was very faithful in her visits to them. Very little is known about Mr. T. except that he is a skilled plumber who occasionally overindulges in alcohol. Since the boys' return to the home, their mother, a good manager and careful housekeeper, has received public assistance for the support of the family.

Various social agencies which have known the T.'s reported that during the past year Mrs. T. has encouraged Anthony to assume the role of head of the household, somewhat to his displeasure and Angelo's dislike. Anthony became defiant and disdainful in his attitude toward her and whenever she urged him and Angelo to get up in time for school they both refused and quarreled with her. They roamed the streets together, joining forces against her nagging. Leaving the house at noon after a combined breakfast-lunch, they would return late at night, offering no explanation of their activities and resenting her queries.

In an effort to help these boys, the court remanded them to a temporary place of detention and ordered that they receive medical, psychological, and psychiatric examinations there. Neither presented any problem in their relationships with other boys at the shelter either in residence, recreation, or classes. Both were found to be in good physical condition except for dental caries. On the Bellevue-Wechsler scale Anthony scored an I.Q. of 96, indicating average intelligence, although in educational tests his ratings showed slight retardation. Marked manipulative dexterity was exhibited. Throughout the psychometric study and in psychiatric interviews, he was cooperative, friendly and spontaneous. No neurotic or psychotic trends were observed, although Anthony expressed hostility toward his father on the basis of what he has been told by his mother. He pictured his mother as an excitable, nervous person who often had to be calmed down. Anthony expressed a rather immature eagerness to heed his mother's admonition to be the "man of the family" by seeking the company of older boys, envying their greater amount of spending money, wishing to be as well clothed, feeling he could boss his younger brothers, and leave household tasks to them. It was recommended that he be placed on probation and encouraged to complete his vocational course. Counseling service for Mrs. T. was suggested to help her reduce her pressures upon Anthony.

Angelo was found to have high average intelligence, with an I.Q. of 110 on the Bellevue-Wechsler scale, but educationally retarded to a serious degree, due mainly to his prolonged absence from school. During psychiatric interviews he was friendly and responsive. No psychotic or neurotic trends were observed; his truancy was felt to be a reaction to inadequate supervision and maternal nagging and preference for Anthony. Through his discussions with Mrs. T. and Angelo, the examining psychiatrist concluded that she was well intentioned but inadequate and therefore recommended that Angelo be placed in an institution for normal boys where he would lead a more regularized life. Neither opposed this plan and the court committed Angelo to an institution having a fine remedial program, where he has made a good adjustment. Anthony was placed on probation and has responded well. Pressure upon him has lessened somewhat as Mrs. T. is utilizing counseling service from a family service agency.

Prognosis for Angelo is favorable, for his is a relatively stable personality. He will be helped to develop wholesome patterns and with maturity will be better able to cope with his mother. It is expected that Anthony also is unlikely to come before the court again as pressure on him lightens.

Placement Needed

LOUIS A.

Louis, 14, a pupil in the 8A grade, is the eldest of three siblings whose father has been unemployable for more than ten years because of abdominal, spleen, and hernia disorders. When Louis was 5 his father developed a manic-depressive psychosis for which he was hospitalized, treated, and then discharged as cured. Family members deny that he has shown any disordered behavior since that time. Mrs. A., obese and lethargic, displays little interest in either her children or her apartment, which is dirty and cluttered. Spending most of her time reading comic books and munching sweets, she allows them to sleep mornings, remain at home during the afternoons, and on the streets at night. When they get into difficulties at school or in the neighborhood, she shrugs her shoulders and does not wish to be bothered. For the past ten years the household has been supported by means of public assistance.

As a result of his truancy and misconduct in class, including the brandishing of a homemade gun, Louis was referred to the court. A year previously, following an outburst of violence, he had been seen at Bellevue Hospital Psychiatric Division whose doctors had advised his parents to leave him there for a brief period of observation, but they refused, rendering it impossible for a diagnosis to be made. After reviewing the facts, the court remanded Louis to Bellevue for observation. There he was found to be in good physical condition and achieved a dull normal I.Q. of 83 in psychometric tests. On the adolescent ward he associated mainly with older, more aggressive boys and was often defiant and quarrelsome, particularly at night when the doctors were not present. No neurotic or psychotic traits were manifested, and the examining psychiatrists recommended that he be placed on probation for an interval, adding that if he continued to truant and to misbehave, he should be placed in an institution for normal boys where he could have a chance to lead a wholesome life.

When probation proved unsuccessful due to Louis' unfavorable home conditions, he was placed in accordance with the hospital's suggestions. Reports from the institution disclosed that he is making a satisfactory adjustment, responding well to supervision and a strong program of sports and farm work coupled with studies.

It is apparent that lax parental supervision in an atmosphere of disinterest and sluggishness precluded Louis' adequate adjustment while he remained at home, for he had no opportunity to develop constructive habits of regularity and effort; therefore, his chance for improvement lay in a placement geared to his needs, and it was fortunate that one was available at a crucial time.

ARTURO A.

Arturo, 15 and enrolled in the 7A grade, has two older brothers, one of whom is unemployed and given to loitering on street corners and the other is an inmate of a state school for mental defectives. After a career as a gunman for a notorious gang, their father was imprisoned two years ago to serve a life sentence on a conviction of homicide. When this occurred, Mrs. A., dull and suspicious, moved the family into a different neighborhood and started to work in a factory. Fearing that other members of the gang or their relatives may seek to retaliate for Mr. A.'s adverse testimony, she shunned normal contacts, stressing that her boys must live by themselves and not associate with others.

Starting with sporadic episodes of truancy, Arturo has absented himself more and more since his father's imprisonment; in class sessions he was defiant and disobedient. Upon referral to court, the judge ordered that he be studied in a guidance clinic. He was found to be in good physical condition, with low average I.Q. of 90 and scholastically retarded two years in reading and arithmetic. No psychiatric deviation was noted and the recommendation was referral of Mrs. A. to a family case work agency. His truancy was attributed to his feeling of embarrassment at his father's predicament and to a lack of parental supervision. Probation was suggested for Arturo and accepted by the court but proved unsuccessful. His mother resisted agency efforts to help her; it was inferred from her attitude and behavior that she was attempting to shield her sons from all contacts with courts and social agencies because she identified these with her husband's trial and incarceration. Whenever the court tried to reach Mrs. A. it was found she had moved, leaving no new address. Then she was reported to have removed from the state, taking her children with her.

Prognosis here is poor because of the long-standing pattern of antisocial behavior within Arturo's family group. To them illegal and criminal acts are as normal and matter of course as law-abiding conduct is in most families. Mrs. A.'s mistrust renders it impossible to aid her and her sons.

ROSE B.

Rose, 15 and a pupil in the 8A grade, has an older sister and a younger brother. After years of marital friction, their parents separated a decade ago and later were divorced when Mr. B. had a child by another woman. He remarried and has been living in another state with Rose's sister and brother. At the time of the separation Rose was placed in an orphanage for a short time until her mother resumed working, when she established a small home for the two of them. Mrs. B. is employed long hours as a bookkeeper, earning a good salary, which she does not hesitate to spend on herself and Rose. Bitterly disappointed in her marriage at 15½, a marriage opposed by her parents because of her extreme youth and that of Mr. B. who was then 17½, Mrs. B. spurned offers of remarriage and was worried that Rose might marry unwisely. Recently Rose's older sister, Grace, returned from her father's household. Being mentally retarded and crippled from infantile paralysis, she is an added responsibility for Mrs. B., who fluctuates in her handling of her daughters. There has been a poor relationship between the sisters; Grace was jealous of Rose's attractiveness and many dates, while Rose resented Grace's having lived for years with their father, who never seemed interested in his younger daughter. By turns Rose has been demanding of her mother and concerned about her.

Until Grace returned, Rose attended school regularly and achieved good grades in all her subjects. Then she began to remain out late at night with her many friends, cut classes, and ceased to be interested in her studies. Poised, with an easy social manner and some insight into her problems, she responded well to counseling in a guidance unit. When her truancy became flagrant, she was referred to the court, which requested reports from the agency where she was known. They had found her to be in good physical condition, of average intelligence, and without emotional disturbance. Their psychiatrist felt that since Rose could not receive adequate supervision while at home and was acting against Grace's presence, a temporary placement would be desirable. Rose was not adverse to the plan and upon remand to an excellent institution, enjoyed the experience of group living. Assisted by a case worker, Rose began to understand her feelings about Grace and about her parents. Upon reaching 16 she was discharged with a favorable prognosis and received an employment certificate.

It is not likely that Rose will become involved in any further delinquency, for she will enjoy working and has been enabled to live at home in more peace and contentment. Despite her father's rejection she is healthy enough emotionally not to have developed any real disturbance over it.

The placement period was a constructive one for her, since she was able to utilize the various forms of help which were available.

KATHERINE D.

Katherine, looking older than her 15 years, and a pupil in the 8B grade, was referred to the court for persistent truancy and misconduct in school such as bullying younger children and taking their pocket money. Resentful of authority and with a precocious interest in sex, she spent most of her time in stores, movies, and dance halls, remaining out until 3 or 4 A.M. An only child whose mother and stepfather were employed long hours, she was disdainful of them and beyond their control. Various conflicting accounts were given of her father—that he had never been married to her mother, that he was dead, that he was living in another state. In any event, there had been no communication with him for over a decade. For most of her life Katherine had lived with her maternal grandmother, Mrs. R., who on her frequent trips South shifted the child to a maternal aunt. Mrs. R. seemed to dislike Katherine, predicting an early death for her, and as soon as her mother remarried sent the girl North.

Mr. and Mrs. D.'s combined earnings from skilled factory work enabled them to maintain a high standard of living. Their apartment was orderly, well furnished, and situated in a good residential section. Mrs. D., hard-working and reticent, felt at a loss in trying to cope with Katherine, giving her an ample allowance and many clothes in an attempt to make up for lack of supervision and guidance. Mrs. D. was reluctant to speak of her own life, implying that she had had a number of highly painful experiences.

In an effort to help Katherine the court had her studied in a mental hygiene clinic, where she was found to be in good physical condition and of normal intelligence, achieving an I.Q. of 98 in the Bellevue-Wechsler scale. No neurotic or psychotic tendencies were elicited, but the prognosis for her adjustment while at home was poor, due primarily to the absence of a constructive routine of living. Accordingly, placement was advised in an institution for normal girls where she would receive close supervision and guidance. This suggestion was accepted by the court, and as soon as a vacancy occurred Katherine was placed in a private institution where her parents contribute to her support. There she has made a somewhat satisfactory adjustment.

Prognosis for Katherine probably will continue to be poor because habits which have been developed over a period of years are not likely to be eliminated in a year or two of placement beginning at the age of 15, especially when the individual is returned to essentially similar home conditions. Of course, Katherine will then be of an employable age, but it is questionable whether she will be willing to work because her mother undoubtedly will continue to give her material possessions in an effort to conciliate her. When she is beyond school age Katherine will be able to use her time as she pleases with little or no restraint.

ARTHUR C.

Arthur, 14 and a pupil in the 8A grade, was referred to the court for excessive truancy. It was learned that he and his family had been known to a private agency for the four preceding years. Their report supplied helpful background data aiding in an understanding of Arthur's problem. He was the eldest of five siblings whose mother, frail and worn, had been seriously ill with pulmonary tuberculosis during the last six years; it was arrested at present but the outlook was not good. For a time she had been hospitalized but had departed against the doctors' advice because she had been troubled about her family. During her illness the four children then living had been placed in institutions for two years. Recently she had a serious gynecologic operation and since then has been too weary to cope with Arthur. During most of their married life Mr. C., although conscientious, has never earned more than a marginal income as an unskilled worker for the city. Even a minimum family budget is curbed by his wages. Constant debts and upsets affecting the family's health as well as their adjustment to each other have been a commonplace for the C.'s, since there were no other employable members to supplement their income and charitable contributions did not suffice or were not always available. Under these pressures Mr. C. deserted on one occasion when his wife was in the hospital, but he returned soon afterward and then was inducted into military service. It was not easy for Mrs. C. to manage during the time of his service, which ended very recently, when he resumed his former employment.

Just before his appearance in court the private family agency had arranged for Arthur's examination in a mental hygiene clinic where he was found to be in good physical condition except for carious teeth, of average intelligence with an I.Q. of 95, and of normal personality. However, because of his well established pattern of truancy, coupled with his mother's physical incapacity to supervise or guide him and his father's long hours of arduous work permitting little attention to his children, it was recommended that he be placed in a rehabilitative center for normal boys. Before deciding upon placement, the court gave Arthur an opportunity on probation, but this proved unsuccessful; his truancy increased, he kept late hours and there was nobody in the home to help him make a better adjustment. Placement followed in the center suggested by the clinic. Both parents were relieved, for they could not control him and feared that he might become involved in serious delinquency if allowed to remain at home.

Reports from the institution state that Arthur has made great strides in his school work and at athletics. The persons in charge plan to have him continue there until he has learned a skilled trade of his own choosing and reaches employable age. He and his parents are pleased with the plan.

Prognosis for Arthur is good, as he is learning to live a regularized life in a constructive setting. When he returns home he will be able to help his family, whom he loves and who love him. The major cause of his previous misconduct—lack of a good routine and supervision within his home—is not present in his substitute home. With no antisocial patterns and a normal personality, his chances of future adjustment are excellent.

HELEN M.

Helen, 13 and a pupil in the 8A grade, was the younger of two siblings whose mother had died in childbirth and whose father, a prosperous grocer, had remarried three years previously. At first Helen and her brother, Vito, had accepted their stepmother, but when they felt that she was overburdening them with household tasks, they rebelled, Vito by running away to his paternal aunt, Mrs. D., and Helen by truanting and keeping late hours. They believed that Mrs. M. was prejudicing their father against them and that they were no longer welcome at home. Both their father and stepmother were very strict disciplinarians. When Vito enlisted in the army, Helen's unhappiness increased; she begged and pleaded with her father to be allowed to live with her aunt, but he refused, convinced that she should live obediently at home where she received every comfort. As her truancy became flagrant Helen was referred to court.

Attempting to help her, the court referred her to a mental hygiene clinic for study. There she was found to be in excellent physical condition and of average intelligence, with an I.Q. of 95 on the Stanford-Binet scale. Educational tests showed her to be slightly retarded in reading. It was evident in psychiatric interviews that Helen had a normal personality; no neurotic or psychotic traits were observed or elicited, although she was unhappy at the lack of affection from her stepmother who impressed the examiner as an egocentric individual, lacking warmth and possessing little understanding of a child's needs. Helen felt bad that Mrs. M. could never be friendly with Mrs. D., whom both children loved dearly, and disliked their visiting her. Mrs. M. told the psychiatrist that she had suffered two nervous breakdowns in the past year from worrying over Helen's truancy and stubborn pleas to live with Mrs. D. Mrs. M. concluded that the best thing to do would be to enroll Helen in a convent school. Throughout the discussion Mrs. M. displayed no affection for either Helen or Vito.

The clinic recommended that Helen be removed from her home and that if Mr. M. persisted in his unwillingness to have her live with his sister, where Helen could obtain affection and security, then she should be placed in a boarding school. At the second court hearing Mr. M. was adamant in his insistence that Helen live at home; he felt that his sister, Mrs. D., would not be strict enough with Helen and she would "get into trouble"; it would be a disgrace to the family for a young daughter not to reside with her father, who kept a nice home for her and was able and willing to provide her with anything she needed. Mrs. D., warm and affectionate, as well as intelligent and alert, pleaded to have custody of Helen, promised to treat her as one of her own daughters. When called upon to express herself, Helen told the judge she wanted to remain at home; she seemed apprehensive of being sent to an institution if she implied any unwillingness to live with her father and stepmother. The court then decided to place her on probation and told Mr. M. to take her home with him. Her attendance record would be followed and if she truanted again, she would be brought back to court.

The question arises whether it would have been advisable to allow Helen to live with her aunt for a trial period. She appeared afraid to express her real preference at the hearing, although she had at the clinic and in office interviews with the court's social workers. There may be the danger that, in trying to conform to accepted behavior standards regarding attendance and evening hours in an atmosphere of rejection and insecurity, she would be repressing her desires and impulses in a manner destructive to mental health. After a period of repression she may perhaps "explode" in more serious delinquency. It seems plain that her stepmother's negative attitude toward Helen will not change and Mr. M. undoubtedly is influenced by his wife's attitude. In the writer's opinion the prognosis for Helen's adjustment is therefore poor.

ENID S.

Enid, 15 and a pupil in the 8B grade, is the youngest of four siblings and the only one of them remaining at home. Because of persistent school absences she was referred to the court, and after a study of the family background a neglect petition was taken. Up to the time her father enlisted in the army a year ago, Enid's school record was good. Despite his sternness and severity, all the children loved him and missed him a great deal. He had worked steadily as a truck driver, and although his earnings had not been large he had managed to provide comfortably for the household. Since his departure Mrs. S., who before her marriage had had a child out of wedlock by another man and who was careless and erratic in her behavior, began to engage in extramarital relationships with men of different races whom she entertained in her home. As this continued she resented Enid's presence, scolded her for minor infractions and beat her whenever she stayed out late at night.

As an aid to the court in planning for Enid, she was examined in a mental hygiene clinic. Except for carious teeth she was found to be in good physical condition, and in psychometric tests she was classified as of low average intelligence with an I.Q. of 89 on the Stanford-Binet scale. She cooperated, but her effort was superficial and careless. Her scholastic achievement showed one year's retardation in arithmetic and reading. During psychiatric discussions Enid was seen to be of normal personality but concerned about her mother's misconduct and rejection. Starting with one or two days of school absence when her father left, Enid gradually developed into a habitual truant as her mother did not encourage her to attend school and no one seemed to notice whether or not she was attending. When interviewed at the clinic Mrs. S. revealed a complete rejection of Enid, but because of a need to be regarded as a good mother refused to consider placement for her child.

The clinic's psychiatrist reported to the court that Enid's home offered so little training and protection that she probably would become involved in serious delinquency if she remained there, and he therefore advised that she be placed in a suitable child-caring institution. Desirable as it was to follow this recommendation, the court was unable to do so because no placement was available for Enid. Public facilities did not exist and the few vacancies within private institutions were being reserved for girls even more in need of protection and care. Although recognizing that it was unwholesome for Enid to continue at home, the court had no alternative. The latest information is to the effect that her truancy has become worse; she has formed a habit of keeping very late hours, attending dance halls and parties, yet there is no way of aiding her while she is at home.

Prognosis for Enid is poor, despite the fact that she is of normal personality, for in the absence of a stable home life her conduct is becoming increasingly worse. It is likely that later she will appear before the court on delinquency charges. Perhaps then she will qualify for a protective placement in a private institution serving girls who have become delinquent. It is tragic that because of lack of placement facilities Enid cannot be helped sufficiently to avoid a delinquent career.

CARL A.

Carl, 14 and enrolled in the 7B grade, has a younger sister, Annette; between them has existed a sense of keen rivalry from the time they were small children. She suffered a serious head injury recently, so that Mrs. A. has become even more concerned and devoted to Annette, much to Carl's discomfiture. Mrs. A., a warm, cheerful individual, has been employed in a garment factory for a year, leaving the house early in the morning and returning late each day except for the times she took off to attend to Annette. By doing her household chores at night, Mrs. A. kept their apartment immaculate. Mr. A., a steam fitter, has been working out of town for the past eight years, coming home week ends too tired to pay attention to his children, who have never learned to know him well. According to his wife Mr. A. is hard-working, set in his ways, and temperate in his habits. She wanted him to obtain a job in the city, but he liked working for his company and did not want to make a change.

When Carl's truancy became chronic and he frequented movies with other lads during school hours, he was referred to court. To secure as complete a picture of him as possible the court referred him to a mental hygiene clinic for study. There he was found to be in excellent physical condition except for carious teeth. In psychometric tests he achieved an I.Q. of 89 on the Stanford-Binet scale, grading with the higher level of the dull normal group. Scholastically he was retarded two years in reading and arithmetic.

During psychiatric interviews he was bored, sulky, and lethargic, partly real and partly assumed. He showed considerable insight into his behavior, was dissatisfied with his mode of life, realized he was wasting his opportunity to acquire an education, but could not bring himself to break off with undesirable companions who truanted regularly. He had a warm relationship with his mother, realized that she was actively interested in him, but provoked her, especially when she compared him with Annette, to his disparagement. Speaking lukewarmly of his father, with whom he has never made friends, Carl expressed disinterest in the week-end visits. No neurotic or psychotic trends were observed and the psychiatrist concluded that Carl had a normal personality but needed more personal interest and training than he could receive at home. With Carl's consent and that of his mother, the clinic suggested that he be placed in a farm school operated by a private religious group.

The court followed this recommendation and Carl was remanded there for a six months' period. With the help of remedial instruction, an active program of sports, farm work and individual counseling, he made such a fine adjustment that the institution was willing to accept him on a full commitment at the expiration of the remand. Both Carl and his mother were pleased with the plan, so a commitment was ordered in view of his progress.

Prognosis for Carl's later adjustment in the communuity appears good, since he has a normal personality and is receiving the guidance and direction he needs. Lack of these was the primary cause of his getting into difficulty rather than an antisocial trend; by the time he is released his habit patterns will be constructive and he will have work skills along with work habits.

LAWRENCE H.

Lawrence, 13 and a pupil in the 6B grade, is the eldest of five siblings whose father, frail and meek, worked as a porter in an office building. Mrs. H., self-effacing and rather lacking in warmth, kept their apartment neat and orderly. It was located within a congested tenement district in the midst of busy traffic. Lawrence, who truanted persistently, was disobedient at home and refused to be moved from his course by either reasoning or punishment. Keeping late hours and roaming the streets, Lawrence preferred the company of older boys who were known in the neighborhood as hoodlums. When he was brought into court as a habitual truant his parents pleaded while he was in another room that he be placed, because they feared he would get into more serious trouble if he continued to live at home; they felt unable to cope with him.

Before making any decision, the court ordered that Lawrence be examined in a mental hygiene clinic. There he was found to be in excellent physical condition except for carious teeth. With an I.Q. of 84 on the Stanford-Binet scale, he was classified as possessing low average intelligence coupled with a definite aptitude for mechanical work, but educationally retarded in the three R's. In psychiatric interviews he was cooperative, pleasant and fairly articulate. He expressed a longing for country life and recalled his pleasure at helping his paternal uncle with farm chores during school vacations. Evincing no neurotic or psychotic tendencies, he was considered to be a boy of normal personality reacting to lack of adequate supervision and to an academic program in advance of his present skills. It was recommended that if possible he be placed with his uncle and enrolled in a rural school.

The clinic's suggestions were discussed with Lawrence, his parents, and uncle. They were pleased and proceeded to make their own arrangements for such a placement after the necessary dental service was obtained. Reports indicate that Lawrence is doing well in a rural school adjacent to his uncle's farm and plans to be a farmer when he grows up.

Prognosis here is good, as Lawrence has no antisocial tendencies and is receiving needed supervision and guidance in a setting which interests him.

JERRY D.

Jerry, 15 and a pupil in the 6A grade, had three older sisters and three younger brothers. Their father, a fatigued, elderly, unskilled laborer who had married three times, died of cancer several years prior to Jerry's first court appearance as a habitual truant. Until Mrs. D. and her eldest daughter, Cornelia, obtained factory work, the family had received financial aid for several years from a private agency, which described the mother as dull and uncooperative. Jerry did not associate with his classmates, preferring the company of older boys who also were truants. In class he was well behaved but seemed to have difficulty in learning. Because of a reading disability Jerry had been referred to a guidance unit of the educational system five years earlier. Repeated psychometric study over this period disclosed a degree of apparent intellectual deterioration. Thus his I.Q. on the Stanford-Binet scale in 1940 was 90, in 1944, 85, and in 1945, 78.

In view of these circumstances the court decided that more intensive study was needed and therefore remanded Jerry to Bellevue Hospital Psychiatric Division for observation. It was important to ascertain whether or not the evident deterioration was caused by an organic involvement. Medical examination revealed that he had a deviated septum, but he was considered too young for plastic repair. A tonsillectomy was advised because of chronic tonsillitis. Ophthalmological tests showed that Jerry had serious astigmatism and glasses were suggested. All neurological tests were negative, so the possibility of a brain disorder was ruled out. He was classified as having borderline intelligence with an I.Q. of 79 on the Stanford-Binet scale. Very serious scholastic retardation was found, because he was a nonreader and his reading achievement was at a 3A level.

No psychiatric deviation was disclosed. He made a good adjustment on the ward and displayed no neurotic or psychotic trend. The examining psychiatrists concluded that Jerry's chief difficulty was an educational one, and since he progressed somewhat with special tutoring in the school within the hospital, they recommended that he be placed on probation and be permitted to continue in their school until the end of the semester. Their advice was followed. However, Jerry participated in three robberies within the succeeding year, acting as the "lookout" each time while his companions robbed small stores at night. Brought before another branch of the court because of these activities, he was again placed on probation and later was transferred to the same court before which he had appeared originally.

Placement was recommended by the court's social service staff, but when Mrs. D. objected it was decided to defer placement and give Jerry another opportunity at home. Essential medical care was secured through the cooperation of hospital authorities.

Prognosis here is poor because Jerry is beyond the control of his mother and his antisocial patterns seem well developed. He needs close supervision and guidance, which he will not receive at home. How effective placement would be is problematical, but at least in a well-rounded group program he would have more of a chance than at home. It is likely that his misconduct will reach such proportions that he will have to be committed to a correctional institution.

MAX N.

Max, 15, and a pupil in the second term of high school, had two younger brothers of whom he was very fond. When Max was 8 his father deserted the home after stormy and prolonged marital friction. After his whereabouts had been unknown to his family for several years, Mr. N. was found to be living in a bigamous marriage with two additional children. He immediately deserted once more and then established a home with a third woman. Generally irresponsible, with an unstable work history, he was rejected by the Army as having a psychopathic personality. Mrs. N., harassed and tired from overwork and emotional strain, has managed to support herself and her sons with the help of Mr. N.'s elderly mother, who has remained friendly to her son's family. Up to a year ago Max had a good scholastic record; then his paternal grandfather, with whom Max had had an excellent relationship, died and Max felt bereft. He became a persistent truant, frequenting movies, parks, and associating with older truants.

Mrs. N. had taken Max to a child guidance clinic but did not continue because she felt he was improving. Six months later Max came to the same clinic in company with another boy who had been treated there. Max requested help, stating that he was considering leaving home and was truanting almost all of the time. However, he did not come again until he was referred back to the clinic for study after being brought to court for unlawful school absences. There he was found to be in good physical condition and of superior intelligence, with an I.Q. of 116 on the Stanford-Binet scale. No educational retardation was revealed. In psychiatric interviews Max was seen to have a normal personality but a conflicted attitude about his father. His habit of truancy was attributed to the lack of a stable home life.

Placement in a rehabilitative center operated by the same agency as the clinic was recommended. The court accepted this suggestion and with the consent of both Max and Mrs. N. committed him there. Under a program of individual counseling service, vocational training in the area of Max's choice, and group recreational activities, he has shown marked improvement. Reports indicate that at the rate he is progressing he will be ready for discharge at 16, at which time he will be equipped with work skills and the capacity to live harmoniously in the community.

Prognosis for Max is good, since he has no antisocial patterns and is obtaining a constructive experience in group living and is accessible to help.

Placement Not Needed

PAUL T.

Paul, 15, and enrolled in the 7A grade, was the youngest of six siblings and the only one remaining at home. His older brothers were in the armed forces and his only sister, Mildred, 20, left the house six months previously after a quarrel with their father when she remained out late at night. From the time Paul was 2 his mother has been a patient in a state hospital for the mentally ill with a diagnosis of manic-depressive psychosis following her premature menopause. Occasionally his father forces Paul to accompany him on visits to Mrs. T., much to Paul's distress at his mother's maniacal excitement. Until he was 8 Paul was cared for by a paid housekeeper; then Mildred took over the household duties but resisted the burden of caring for him. However, the older brothers helped, particularly Otto, to whom Paul became attached. Since Otto's departure six months ago, Paul began truanting excessively, sleeping in the mornings, preparing a sketchy noon meal, and roaming about the streets during the afternoons.

Mr. T., a hard-working carpenter, strict and devoted to his children, felt bad when Paul was referred to court as a habitual truant. Mr. T. pleaded that Paul was a good boy who had fallen into bad habits because there was no one at home to supervise him. Expressing sorrow at Mildred's leaving home, Mr. T. regretted that he had been so strict with her and longed for her return. He hoped that Otto would be released from the army soon to help Paul, who always listened to Otto and followed his suggestions. Their father impressed the court as a stable, intelligent person who wanted to do his utmost for Paul but was handicapped seriously by the lack of a mother in the household.

In an attempt to assist Paul, the court remanded him to a temporary detention home and ordered that he be examined there. The medical report was negative, indicating good physical condition. He was classified as possessing average intelligence, with an I.Q. of 95 on the Bellevue-Wechsler scale. Scholastic retardation was evidenced in both reading and arithmetic. In psychiatric interviews he was quiet but amiable in manner, alert and responsive. No neurotic or psychotic patterns were disclosed. Paul expressed a definite feeling of need for his mother, and despite his fears of her excitement, he desired her home. Speaking at length of Otto, whom he missed greatly, he admitted that he had become habituated to truancy because Otto was no longer there to see that he arose in time to attend school or to make sure that he did his homework. If Mildred were home, she would help him "to do the right thing." As it was, his father went to work early in the morning, returning late in the evening, and in the time between there was nobody to notice what Paul was or was not doing. It was felt that with supervision in the home he would be able to make an adequate adjustment.

The court thereupon sent for Mildred, a calm, intelligent person, discussed the whole matter with her and requested her help. She related that she had been wanting to return but had hesitated, hoping her father would beg her to do so. She seemed glad at the opportunity to return, as did her father and Paul. Mr. T. made arrangements to work nearer his house so that he could relieve Mildred somewhat. Otto was expected back shortly, and it was believed that his presence would be a stabilizing influence. Paul's attendance record improved steadily and therefore he was discharged from probation.

Prognosis is good because neither Paul nor his family have antisocial patterns and the members are closely knit and helpful to him.

JOAN C.

Joan, 14 years of age and a pupil in the 8B grade, was the second of five siblings whose parents had a good marital relationship and were affectionate toward them. The family, whose members were attached to one another, occupied a five-room apartment in an old tenement building within a congested delinquency area. Mr. C. was employed steadily as a skilled laborer, while his wife worked late afternoons and evenings as a hospital attendant. During her absence from home, Agnes, the elder daughter, 17, supervised the younger children and prepared dinner. All the children had excellent school records until the last semester when Joan, becoming very friendly with an older truant, Constance, began remaining away from afternoon sessions, although her behavior in classes, at home and in the neighborhood continued to be good. As Joan's truancy continued she lost interest in school subjects, neglected her homework and displayed little effort.

Unknown to their parents, Constance and Joan spent many of their afternoons at movies and many evenings at dances. Finally they disappeared from a school dance and after several weeks of intensive search, during which Mr. and Mrs. C. were frantic with worry, both girls were found working as waitresses in another state and residing in a rooming house. When they were returned to the city they were brought before the court and remanded temporarily to a shelter while undergoing medical, psychological, and psychiatric tests. Joan was found to be a precociously developed adolescent with impaired vision due to a congenital uncorrected internal squint, or strabismus. Since the squint by this time had almost corrected itself surgery was not advised, although the damage to her vision was irreparable, but glasses were imperative. Other medical findings were essentially negative.

In psychometric and psychiatric examinations Joan was most cooperative and friendly. She achieved an I.Q. of 89 on the Stanford-Binet scale, but her score was not considered to reflect accurately her native endowment, as she was worried by her escapade and failed to function efficiently. The psychologist concluded that Joan possessed average intelligence. No indication of emotional disturbance was evidenced in the Rorschach pattern. The psychiatrist confirmed previous social evaluation that Joan came from a stable, closely knit family of good standards and strong ties. Joan had had a misunderstanding with Agnes and consequently had refused to accept her supervision. Truancy had become a pleasurable habit shared with Constance, and before Joan realized how far she was going she had acceded to the out-of-state adventure. Deeply sobered by her detention, repentant and truthful, she asked for a chance to rehabilitate herself at home and at school. Fond of her family, she wept at the anxiety she had caused her parents and siblings, who had missed her daily, and promised that she would not associate with Constance or her companions, who were all older than Joan. No neurotic or psychotic trends were evidenced, so a diagnosis of normal personality was made with a recommendation that she be placed on probation with closer supervision in the home.

At the expiration of the remand period, the psychiatrist's advice was discussed with Joan and her family, who were overjoyed to be together again. She was placed on probation; Mrs. C. shifted her working hours to permit better supervision of Joan and the younger children, and the parents accepted the court's suggestion that they move to a better neighborhood. Joan's improvement was such that probation was not needed more than a three-month period. She graduated from the elementary grades and entered the high school of her choice, where her attendance, behavior, and scholarship were highly satisfactory.

Prognosis is good primarily because the major reason for Joan's misconduct was a lack of sufficient supervision, susceptible of easy correction in a favorable home setting with stable, affectionate, and adequate parents and a child of normal personality.

NANCY M.

Nancy, 15½, and a pupil in the first term of high school, was referred to the court as a habitual truant. Several years before her mother's death of cancer two years ago, her father had deserted his family and has continued to live with the same woman friend, manifesting no interest in his children. Working intermittently at an unskilled job, he never earned enough to support two households and has felt no responsibility for the upkeep of his family, who received relief until the eldest daughter, Bridgit, obtained employment as a stenographer. Since Mrs. M. died, Mary, the next oldest sibling, has kept house for herself, Bridgit, Nancy, and the youngest child, Winifred. Their brother Billy, 10, made his home with his elderly paternal grandparents, who have a tiny apartment and a small income.

Up to the time of Mrs. M.'s death, Nancy had a good school record in attendance, conduct, and scholarship, but ever since then has been truanting at an accelerating rate until she was absent a whole semester. In company with older girls she frequents movies and department stores, at one time leaving her home to live with a girl in a furnished room. While with her family Nancy has been cynical and defiant, resenting Mary's supervision. When asked by the court why she was truanting, Nancy replied that she was ashamed to attend classes in which the other girls were much smaller than she; first she had been absent a few days at a time, then, when nothing had been done about it, she remained out a week at a time, increasing this to several weeks and months when she found she "could get away with it."

After a period of probation proved unsuccessful, the court remanded Nancy to a temporary shelter and ordered that she be studied in the court's clinic. She was found to be well nourished and well developed, much above average in height and weight, in excellent physical condition. In psychometric tests she was classified as having average intelligence with an I.Q. of 99. It was felt that she could have achieved a higher I.Q. had she exerted herself. During psychiatric interviews she was cooperative, a little timid, not spontaneous. No neurotic or psychotic trends were disclosed, and it was concluded that her personality was normal. After her mother's death she had drifted into a pattern of truancy when she found that she could absent herself without penalty. Now she was awaiting her sixteenth birthday when she could obtain an employment certificate and a job which would enable her to buy nice clothes. Later she planned to marry and have a home of her own. It was the psychiatrist's opinion that probation should be tried once more, because placement was not indicated. He felt that as soon as Nancy was permitted to work there would be no further difficulty with her.

Accordingly, the court again placed Nancy on probation, realizing that her disinterest in school and her desire to work for pretty clothes, which could not be supplied to her by the family, would mitigate against her regular attendance in the few remaining months of the school year. Her habit of remaining away from classes was too well developed to be overcome in such a short period of time under the same circumstances, but placement was inadvisable. She made an effort to attend but, as expected, the number of days present was exceeded by the days absent. Finally she secured her work permit and liked her sales-clerk job.

Prognosis here is good because Nancy is a stable girl of normal intelligence and personality who in the light of her rapid physical development was more satisfied to work than to continue at school with smaller classmates. Her truancy should have received attention long before it did. The question arises: Should not Nancy have been allowed a work permit before her sixteenth birthday? For her it might have been more constructive than to attempt forcing her back to school under the circumstances. However, some educators argue that to reward truancy with an opportunity to work would stimulate additional truancy rather than prevent it.

GUIDO R.

Guido, 15 and a pupil in the 8A grade, was the youngest of four siblings whose parents were congenial and affectionate. Mr. R., a bricklayer, intelligent, industrious and deeply interested in his family, admitted to a visiting teacher that lately he and Mrs. R., also intelligent, alert and an excellent homemaker, have been overindulgent with Guido, letting him do as he pleased. Ever since their two eldest sons have been serving overseas, the parents have been so anxious about them that they have relaxed their supervision of Guido, the only remaining son. Taking advantage of their preoccupation, he began staying out late at night, then was too tired to get up in time for school, slept late, and then wandered about the streets enjoying his new freedom. Soon the habit became so strong that he did not want to go to school at all and began associating with older truants. At this point he was referred to court as a habitual truant.

Mr. and Mrs. R. were aghast at being summoned to court with Guido, for it was the first time there had been any difficulty with their children. They had not realized the extent to which Guido had been absenting himself from classes. He could scarcely believe that anything would be done, inasmuch as his activities had escaped notice for over eight months. His attitude was that there was much ado about nothing. Deciding to assist Guido in recognizing the seriousness of his behavior, the court remanded him to a temporary place of detention while undergoing study. In excellent physical condition, of average intelligence and normal personality, Guido made a fine adjustment there after the first day. Pleasant, active and helpful, he wanted to be home but made the best of the situation in which he found himself. The examining psychiatrist helped Guido to see that it was advisable for him to slough off his habit of truancy and replace it with the more realistic habit of regular school attendance. In discussions with Mr. and Mrs. R. they were helped to understand that Guido needed their supervision and guidance; without these he could become involved in serious trouble as well as grow up without an education. Their worry about their elder sons was understandable but was having an adverse effect upon Guido, one that his brothers would not approve. The parents promised to abide by the psychiatrists' advice and pleaded for Guido's return to the home.

Probation was recommended and accepted by the court to the satisfaction of Guido and his parents, who were referred to a private family agency for counseling service. He returned to school, graduated into the vocational high school of his choice, where he made a highly creditable record. Since it was no longer necessary to continue him on probation, he was discharged.

Prognosis is good for Guido, since the chief causal factor in his misconduct was a temporary lack of supervision and guidance by adequate parents having the capacity and willingness to help him become a mature adult.

PETER W.

Peter, 9, a pupil in the 3A grade, was referred to court as a persistent truant. He spent his time playing around the school building with undesirable companions or roaming the streets accompanied by other children. On one occasion he was found by a policeman at midnight on a well-lighted corner. Ill-clothed, unkempt and thin, Peter presented a pathetic appearance. He was the eldest of six children, the only one born of a relationship with Mr. O., with whom Peter lived for a brief period during the previous year. His half siblings were born of a union between Mr. and Mrs. W., who after living together for eight years found that their unrecorded marriage was void. This had been discovered when Mrs. W. applied for a government allowance provided for the wives of servicemen. Since she felt that he had not treated her well, had gambled, and had not supported her properly, she decided not to legalize her union with Mr. W. as he desired, but instead married Mr. S., whom she had met recently. He, too, was in the armed services, and she believed that he would be a good father to all her children.

Mr. W. was upset by her decision and several times asked social agencies to investigate her home to see if his children were receiving good care. They found that despite her employment as a domestic and consequent absence from the household for part of each day, she kept the younger children neat, clean, and well nourished. She seemed less interested in Peter. As soon as she received a government allotment as Mr. S.'s wife, she gave up her job and supervised the children more carefully.

When the court asked Mrs. W., or Mrs. S., as she was later called, about Peter, she responded that she had had her hands so full with her younger children and her former job that she had not been able to give him proper care. She promised to do better, expressing a degree of warmth and affection for him. Evidently the marital surprise was a shock to her, but she felt that she had pursued a wise course in ridding herself of Mr. W. and marrying Mr. S. She told of the latter's liking for all of her children and was convinced that he would be kind and helpful to them as well as to her.

In an effort to assist Peter, the court ordered that he be studied in its clinic. He was found to be undernourished but otherwise in good physical condition. In psychometric tests he was cooperative, concentrated well, scored an I.Q. of 98, denoting average intelligence, but was unable to read, indicating severe scholastic retardation attributed mainly to his excessive absences. During psychiatric interviews Peter was bright, alert, poised, and showed himself to be intelligent and observant in his responses to questions. No psychotic or neurotic traits were evidenced, although he expressed some concern because his father was not in the home. Peter had developed the habit of truanting while his mother had been away from home at her job. Since she had stopped working two months ago he had thought of attending school again but had not realized its importance and had kept postponing his return. Now that he and his mother had been brought to court, he knew that he must go to school, and she would see to this.

Probation was recommended by the clinic and ordered by the court, who cautioned Mrs. S. upon the necessity for her giving Peter adequate supervision and guidance. As she became more alert to his activities, his attendance improved markedly and he was discharged from probation within six months. A program of remedial instruction in reading is proving beneficial to him.

In spite of the curious marital picture, prognosis is good for Peter, since Mrs. W. loves her children, has stable traits, and knows now that her supervision and guidance are as essential for Peter as for her other children and that the major reason for his misconduct was the lack of such care. What the situation will be when Mr. S. returns remains to be seen.

Chapter VII

A CHALLENGE TO COMMUNITY ORGANIZATION

CHILD OFFENDERS present a distinct challenge to community organization, both in respect to the causal elements responsible for their predicaments and the treatment methods and facilities required for their rehabilitation and care. As individuals and as members of family groups most of them can be helped successfully to take their places as productive members of society. To ignore or to minimize this truth is not only shortsighted but cruel and extremely wasteful.

With thoughtful community planning and concerted action based upon expert knowledge and understanding, plus the courage to admit existing lacks in our social service and educational structures, a considerable proportion of juvenile delinquency can be prevented. Instead of the piecemeal stopgaps so often encountered, unified improvements which reflect an appreciation of overall needs are essential.

To our shame, those of us most familiar with the facts through daily attempts to assist children enmeshed in the law's intricacies and delays have stood silently by, leaving to those less informed the task of calling public attention to the problems involved. Under these circumstances it is not at all surprising that various panaceas are offered, each purporting to be the final answer. Among those given wide publicity are slum clearance, recreation programs, compulsory lecture series for wayward parents, and most recently, the sentencing of neglectful parents to jail for contributing to the unlawful conduct of their children.

That better housing, recreation, and parental education are of value no one can gainsay. Yet the fact remains that often those children most in need of supervised play seldom frequent playgrounds and community houses and rarely join such organizations as police athletic leagues, Boy Scouts, or Girl Scouts. Hence they are not reached by recreational programs.

When parents can participate in voluntary parental education, there is more likelihood that they will be receptive to its teachings than when they are forced to attend. Those parents who need it most usually are unaware of their need and unreceptive or emotionally unable to absorb the instruction given. Pressure and authoritative handling result in increased resentment toward the children whose misbehavior occasioned the compulsory action.

The vogue now being followed by certain judges of sentencing to jail parents who have contributed to the delinquency of their children has its dangerous aspects. When the circumstances are analyzed, it is usually found that these people are themselves "more sinned against than sinning" and require specialized care. The very factors that have brought about their own disintegration and disorganization are again operating to produce maladjustment in their children.

To imprison an offending parent in the hope and expectation that this will deter other parents from contributing to the delinquency of their offspring is a sad reflection upon the caliber of the sentencing judge. When will judges learn that the hoary concept of punishment as a deterrent of crime is fallacious—even pernicious? The history of criminal law and penology demonstrates that punishment not only fails to prevent wrongdoing but tends to lull the public into a mistaken belief that the problem is solved.

A child who is already in trouble and feels bitter about his parent's drunken and disorderly conduct or marital misadventures is even more upset and disturbed when, in addition, his parent is jailed and this becomes known among schoolmates, teachers, and neighbors. The burden of guilt becomes even more onerous when the child realizes that if it were not for his own court appearance his parent would not be in prison. Moreover, relations between these parents and their children become even more strained and destructive than before. To believe that such a course of action prevents further delinquency among them or others is to place one's head in the proverbial sand.

Attacks upon delinquency must be many sided, but the first step is to focus attention upon causation.

Causal Factors

Study of the cases found in the preceding chapters and throughout court records indicates that while there is no single cause of delinquency, the most pervasive element producing misconduct is lack of a stable home life. The question arises: What is a stable home life? It may be defined as one in which there is marital harmony between father and mother, regularity of living with a respect for orderly behavior and fairness, familial affection not equivalent to overindulgence, together with careful supervision and guidance of a child's activities. Religious faith and teaching are powerful supporting elements in achieving family solidarity.

The significance of a disturbed and irregular family life as a cause of youthful misbehavior can hardly be overemphasized. Destructive parental attitudes and patterns which often lead to a "broken home" are found to have a more devastating effect than the absence of one parent from the household. All too frequently, it is not the "broken home" but the personalities and events which led to the disruption of the home that are responsible for the child's misconduct.

Wherever family stability exists there is practically no delinquency, except in rare instances, such as when a child is suffering from an organic brain disease or other mental illness not derived from home conditions and his illness is manifested in behavior disorders, or when a child is so mentally retarded that despite supervision he is led astray by more intelligent youths or adults who exploit his oversuggestibility and his deficiencies in reasoning ability, or when a mentally deficient child has precocious physical development coupled with a lack of sexual control.

Absence of a sound family life may result in personal instability, neurotic traits, neurosis, psychoneurosis, or mental illness, each of which may be exemplified in acts of delinquency. Without adequate supervision, a mentally retarded child or even one of normal intelligence and personality may develop habits of misconduct. Children expertly diagnosed as psychopathic personalities who are known to courts usually come from extremely disorganized homes in which there are grave irregularities of conduct among familial members, due to a combination of hereditary and environmental elements.

It is plain that not every child whose home life is without stability will become a delinquent, but his chances of developing an integrated personality are fewer than for others. That he may do so despite highly adverse circumstances is illustrated in Chapter VI. Amid destructive family conditions, some children develop normally; they seem to have an inner resiliency or strength sufficient to combat these negative influences.

However, habitual truancy even among children of normal personality, caused mainly by a lack of adequate supervision, may grow into more serious misconduct in association with other delinquents, who engage first in truancy, then in petty thefts, and graduate to major offenses when their first ventures into crime are uncurbed.

Children who are left unsupervised are prone to get into difficulties, especially when they know that their parents are not particularly interested in what is happening. Many youthful offenders have expressed deep resentment of their parents' disinterest and failure to be companionable in and out of the home.

During the war years, when a high proportion of mothers were employed, a number of children who were normal in every respect became delinquent through an absence of parental supervision. Frequently their mothers were unaware of anything amiss until the court notified them of pending charges. Some were vastly indignant; others were humiliated and chagrined.

Adequate supervision presupposes parents who are not too dull or disturbed to realize its importance, who are sufficiently interested in their children's activities, who spend a normal amount of time at home, especially in the mornings, after school hours, and at night, or provide a suitable substitute (one who is competent and has warmth of feeling), and who are able to give constructive direction and guidance.

From their earliest years, children require and usually welcome a regular routine of living if it is not too rigid and is accompanied by affection. Many parents are unaware of its importance and do not realize that a program of routinized living in itself gives security to a child and helps him to develop good habits and emotional balance.

Physical defects are another potent causal agent. When, unknown to their parents, children are suffering from impaired hearing or vision, enlarged and diseased tonsils, or dental caries adversely affecting their vitality, the rate of truancy mounts alarmingly. Unable to compete on equal terms with their classmates because of such handicaps, these youngsters remain away from school, frequently for prolonged periods. During these intervals, many drift into association with older delinquents and additional criminal careers are begun.

Even when they return to school, these offenders are behind in their studies, and with a continuation of curable defects, they again truant to escape from almost unbearable strains. Timely medical care could be made available with a minimum of intelligent effort. That is the tragic but hopeful aspect of this particular causal element.

Scholastic retardation is also found to precipitate delinquent behavior in a substantial number of instances. Almost invariably, habitual truants receive low scores in reading and arithmetic tests, even those who possess good learning ability. To avoid confusion, one should bear in mind that lack of normal educational achievement is not necessarily due to mental deficiency. Clinical studies disclose that in many cases it is attributable to emotional dysfunctioning brought about by individual and family difficulties which require skilled attention. At other times, low achievement scores result from physical illness or defect, from poor study habits, or from disinterest in classwork occasioned by lack of variety in subject matter to meet the requirements of children who have little capacity or interest in academic subjects.

The more disinterest that is felt, the higher the ratio of school absences and the more marked the retardation becomes, with a consequent increase in maladjustment. It assumes the proportions of a vicious circle. Efforts to mold all elementary pupils into a setting of academic learning cause school dissatisfactions and frustrations. These find expression in socially undesirable behavior among the large dull normal group as well as among those in lower intellectual levels.

While insufficient facilities for remedial instruction add to the problem, such teaching is not alone the solution, because most of these pupils do not attend classes consecutively enough to profit much from special help in reading and arithmetic.

In failing to offer more realistic curricula in elementary and junior high schools, more individual medical and psychological examinations, together with skilled counseling services and more individual attention in less crowded classes, the schools are stimulating the high incidence of juvenile delinquency so prevalent in both urban and rural communities.

Diagnosis

As in other fields, diagnosis in cases of juvenile delinquency has far outstripped treatment. Yet much remains to be done in refining the diagnostic process and making it more generally available. Its usefulness will grow as expertness increases and is more readily understood by parents, educators, courts, social agencies, and child-caring institutions by means of patient and detailed interpretation.

Sound treatment is based upon prompt, full, and accurate study, for any plan which does not rest upon such a foundation is but a patchwork and usually fails to achieve a lasting improvement. When one attempts to treat delinquency in a child without knowing why he misbehaves, it is like a doctor treating symptoms rather than the disease itself.

Naturally, in many instances temporary treatment may accompany even preliminary diagnosis, just as a doctor may take immediate action to alleviate painful or uncomfortable symptoms while proceeding to have laboratory tests made which may prove essential to a complete diagnosis.

Social workers and physicians are confronted daily with the fact that the dividing line between diagnosis and treatment is often vague and uncertain. Both may be merged from the start of a case. At times it is imperative to give immediate care, as, for example, when a court resorts to a temporary remand of a child to protect him from vicious surroundings. Simultaneously, arrangements can be made to have him studied clinically to ascertain the nature and extent of his problem and how best to assist him.

Diagnosis begins with social study of the child in his family setting. It is axiomatic that the earlier this process is begun, the greater is the opportunity for effective help. In essence, it is a casework function demanding as high a degree of training and skill as that required for an intake interviewer in a progressive agency. Accurate analysis at the start precludes the many futile efforts that are encountered so frequently between the first misconduct and later court appearances.

One reason why habitual truancy is often the beginning of a delinquency career is that expert study is not given truants at the inception of their chronic absences. Clinical findings reveal that the same factors which led to poor attendance records persisted unnoticed and were responsible for the later, graver offenses.

Systematic referral methods and maximum use of social service exchange data are as valuable to social workers within schools, attendance offices, and courts, as in family agencies. Any such tool aids the worker in understanding the child she is attempting to help. A child's school record of attendance, health, achievement, and behavior, together with accounts of home visits made by truant officers or other workers, cast further illumination and facilitate the sifting process.

The more pertinent information that is thus available, the more readily an adequate plan for the child can be formulated. Yet some attendance officers and supervisors remain unaware of the importance of social data, and it is a struggle to persuade them to obtain social service exchange reports and other enlightening material.

The School Part of the New York City Children's Court found it advisable to supply specific referral forms to other groups and to organize definite referral procedures so that there would be an orderly flow of cases. While referral policies and methods must be geared to agency capacities, nevertheless these may be used to stimulate improvements in social service practice.

Interviews, both individual and group, together with conferences complete the preliminary diagnostic period.

After the social and educational information is at hand and the discussions mentioned above have taken place, the next step is that of evaluation and a determination of the implications. From these a tentative plan can be developed. Consultation services are of major importance here, since various kinds of skills and experience can contribute toward accurate diagnosis. In the evaluative process, the psychiatric social worker who possesses clinical and educational experience has a valuable role. He is in a position to assist other workers in concluding whether or not medical, psychological, psychiatric examinations, or all three are indispensable for a particular child or adult, and if so, where these should be made.

For full diagnosis of a child's difficulties the social study must be supplemented by these examinations. Whether the child should be tested privately, in a clinic, or while hospitalized depends upon a variety of factors. So does the issue of whether the studies should be made while the child remains at home or is placed temporarily in a foster home, a shelter, or in another type of institution.

For effective results, it is vital to develop cooperative policies and procedures for the transmission and use of significant data and for the presence of the parties concerned at scheduled times and places.

Experience indicates that the single, most important element is that the examinations be conducted by competent personnel, trained and experienced in administering tests and interpreting their findings. They are able to take into account organic and constitutional factors affecting the patient, as well as the social and functional aspects of the problem.

Wherever an educational system is equipped with such facilities as exist in the Bureau of Child Guidance of the New York City Board of Education, it is usually preferable to utilize these if their intake permits. There is less apprehension and less stigma attaching to examinations within the educational framework. Hence there is more acceptance on the part of parents. Moreover, these clinics are more conversant with school problems and special educational resources than hospital clinics or private practitioners.

Of vital significance in these examinations is the teamwork of social caseworker, physician, psychologist, and psychiatrist, who pool their knowledge of the child and unify their findings in a comprehensive report.

Other guidance centers, hospital and court clinics also provide useful examination service. All these groups are sadly understaffed and overloaded with work. This means that they tend to become primarily centers for diagnosis, with less and less time for treatment. Yet they are unable to accept many referrals even for study.

On occasion clinical examinations disclose the probability of serious emotional disturbance, making advisable twenty-four hour a day observation and the use of equipment such as the electro-encephalogram machine, which is found only in a psychiatric hospital. More conclusive findings can then be made. There then arises the issue of voluntary versus involuntary admissions to a hospital for psychiatric observation.

A child may be admitted into a psychiatric hospital either when his parent gives written consent or upon a court order termed a remand or remand commitment. The first method is voluntary, with an implication that the parent may remove his child at any time in agreement with or against the advice of the hospital authorities.

On the other hand, entrance under a court order is compulsory, and the child must remain for a specified time unless the court order is changed or overruled. A remand means that at the expiration of the observation period the child must be returned to the court issuing the remand. There a further decision will be made concerning the offender.

Where there is a remand commitment, the hospital officials may bring the patient into a special term of another court and ask that he be committed to a state institution for the mentally ill or to a school for the mentally deficient, if their findings warrant such action. In New York City a special term of the Supreme Court is located within the Psychiatric Divisions of Bellevue and Kings County Hospitals to hear these cases and those of adult patients alleged to be mentally ill or feeble-minded, and recommendations are made for state institutional care.

A single observation period may extend from a few days to thirty days, and additional observation may be ordered if recommended. Thirty days is the customary interval for child offenders, as this usually offers sufficient opportunity for comprehensive psychiatric and psychological study as well as thorough medical and neurological examinations. Each patient's behavior receives detailed scrutiny and notation.

The School Part of the New York City Children's Court has adopted a policy of not going forward with such remand proceedings until after an outpatient clinic has officially recommended a period of hospitalization on the basis of its findings. The only exception made is where the child or parent, when brought before the court, is so obviously in need of immediate observation as to preclude an outpatient study.

This court also utilizes remand commitments rather than remands in observation cases to obviate repetitious hearings and harmful delays.

The subject of voluntary versus involuntary hospitalization of a child warrants comment. A fundamental principle of social service is that an individual's participation in planning and action is vital and should be encouraged. But when a parent is confronted with the probability of mental illness or marked mental deficiency in his child, he is likely to be overwhelmed and to deny that the condition exists. He needs the authoritative but understanding help of the court as an opportunity to share his responsibility.

Hospital records are replete with examples in which a parent has expressed his willingness by signing voluntary admission papers only to demand his child's immediate release under pressure from the child, other relatives, and a parental burden of guilt. No comprehensive observation was possible because of the patient's premature departure against the advice of hospital personnel.

A parent's fears and anxieties about his child's entrance into an observation ward are understandable and considerable reassurance should be offered. Certain judges also have these feelings of trepidation and express fears that the experience will prove harmful to the child, even though competent psychiatrists in a guidance clinic or court clinic have stated that observation was urgent. These fears and anxieties are not allayed but intensified by distorted tales of occurrences within hospitals.

It is not easy to reassure either judges or parents on this score when they realize that other children who already are ward patients are there because of manifestations of psychiatric disturbance and that their behavior is not normal. Close supervision of these patients is imperative, and separate children's wards are indispensable.

Most of the dissatisfaction that is voiced stems from cases in which adolescent patients became violent and, in the absence of special facilities, were shifted to adult wards. That special facilities do not exist is truly deplorable and should be remedied without delay. However, it is recognized that appropriations for improvements within public hospitals are exceedingly difficult to obtain. Staff members plead for these, but their pleas receive scant attention from budgetary groups.

Because voluntary admission for observation places an unbearable burden upon parents, the court has to accept responsibility for compulsory action in those cases where there is a firm foundation for hospitalization. Its task is to interpret the need for such action and the resulting benefit to the child offender. The court is in a position to bear the brunt of parental resentment, displeasure, and complaints, for it is clear that these arise from their grief, anxiety, and feelings of responsibility and guilt. To procrastinate for lack of courage is to harm the child, since his condition may become progressively worse and he may become involved in more serious delinquency.

Outpatient study generally can be made while the child remains at home. Conversely, if the home is hazardous, as in cases of incest, gross brutality, or the like, temporary placement must be arranged with provision for clinic attendance. Similar action has to be taken where the parent refuses to have the child attend a clinic, or where he is a chronic runaway or is associating with highly undesirable companions and is beyond parental control.

Whether the temporary placement is in a foster home, shelter, or other child-caring institution, depends upon the child's problem, balanced against available community resources.

Temporary detention in a shelter can be a constructive experience for an offender and also afford opportunity for diagnosis. Whether or not it results in this depends upon the quality of the personnel and presence or absence of diagnostic resources. All too often shelters provide neither, for they are usually indifferently staffed, drab, overcrowded, lacking in clinical facilities, recreational and educational programs. They are geared mainly to custodial care pending judicial hearings.

At one of the most progressive, namely Youth House of

New York City, there is alert leadership, a friendly, understanding atmosphere, planned education and recreation, and the beginnings of a valuable clinical service embracing social casework, psychometric and psychiatric study by well trained, interested practitioners. They furnish the court and social agencies with significant data concerning the problems and potentialities of the boys remanded there. Unfortunately, its insufficiency of staff, together with its antiquated physical structure and lack of outdoor play space prevent Youth House from doing a more effective job.

A unique feature at the present is that, with the aid of public funds, it is operated jointly by private social agencies of various religious faiths. They select the director and are responsible for major policies and practices through an interfaith board. Unlike many places of temporary detention, Youth House makes genuine efforts to interpret its work to the community at large as well as to professional groups.

Arrangements are being made for Youth House to be transferred to the local public welfare authorities as the high quality of its service has been demonstrated and the city officials have finally come to the conclusion that they must accept responsibility for operation of a public detention home for child offenders.

Persistently there has been a feeling that because a child's stay in a detention home is designed to be temporary, there is nothing that can be done for him there except to furnish custodial care until the court disposes of his case. A large number of social workers have never seen the inside of a shelter, and while they are vaguely aware of something amiss, they do not realize that many children linger for months amid stultifying conditions, awaiting court action. Frequently no information is given as to their stay, and the child may depart more set in patterns of misbehavior than when he entered. This is particularly true when neglected children are commingled with delinquents.

Even if a youthful offender spends but a few days or a week in a shelter, his stay can be productive if programs are developed which will be responsive to his needs. The first requisite is the employment of trained caseworkers. Those shelters which cannot add clinical facilities at once can work out arrangements with existing clinics and hospitals for the study of children during the detention period.

Medical, psychometric, and psychiatric reports usually are vital in the diagnostic process, since these enlighten social workers and courts as to underlying causal factors responsible for misconduct and focus attention on what treatment is likely to prove efficacious. Another purpose these reports serve is to provide research data into basic questions of cause and cure in the realm of delinquency and crime.

It is evident that the examiners wish to have the results of their labors used. To help achieve this end for the benefit of child offenders and of society, several criteria are offered as to the form and contents of specialized reports. These are proffered not in a spirit of criticism but as an appeal that the examinations conducted be of maximum usefulness. Comments are based upon scrutiny and discussion of several thousand such reports which were submitted to social agencies and juvenile courts, including those outlined in the preceding chapters.

It is noteworthy that, by and large, medical summaries, aside from neurological, are received with more credence and less skepticism than either psychometric or psychiatric reports. If a physician states that he examined Johnny upon a certain date and found him to be suffering from tuberculosis or congenital syphilis and immediate hospitalization should be arranged for him, no judge is likely to believe that he knows more than the doctor about Johnny's medical condition. On the contrary, the judge is inclined to make his decision in accordance with the medical advice given.

But many judges are prone to feel that they know as much or more about a child or adult than either a psychologist or a psychiatrist, especially if their reports are a morass of obtuse and obscure terminology. In this event, there is a tendency to brush aside both diagnosis and recommendations. With the exception of a few well known experts, the examiners are unknown to courts. Therefore, if their reports have shortcomings, these are not overcome by the signatures.

Since medical summaries, which generally are relatively clear-cut and objective, are easily accepted, there is no necessity to dwell on these except to suggest that highly technical phrases be accompanied by lay terms. Medical dictionaries are not always on hand for immediate translations.

For clarity, psychological reports should always specify the names of the tests used, the scores received on each, any deviation between innate intellectual capacity and performance, the degree of educational retardation, the classification, and the results of the Rorschach test. Interpretive data is helpful, particularly concerning the Rorschach pattern. Factual and interpretive data should be distinct, couched in clear, detailed language and outlined in logical order, with professional terms followed by lay expressions.

Examiners should bear in mind that even today there are many judges who have little or no training in psychology, and some of those who have had are unfamiliar with current psychological trends.

Where a substantial degree of feeble-mindedness is found, the examiner should indicate unmistakably whether or not commitment to a state institution for the mentally deficient is imperative and why. In the absence of a definite recommendation the court will not order such a commitment.

Psychiatric reports are more difficult to prepare, since ordinarily the subject matter is even less familiar to laymen than psychological data. Similar principles are as applicable, i.e., clear, well constructed arrangement of content, both as to findings and advice, with technical phraseology accompanied by a translation into lay terms. Logical sequence is of prime importance in attaining an acceptance of psychiatric summaries.

If hospitalization, placement, or commitment is advocated, the reasons should be stated as explicitly and concretely as possible. Likewise, if parole or probation is advised, the prognosis should be set forth with clarity and notation made as to whether or not treatment should be made available in a clinic or other center.

It is essential that any suggestions made should embody a current awareness of existing community resources, intake policies, programs, strengths, and gaps. Otherwise, the advice lacks practicality. If the most highly desirable form of care is unavailable, that should be indicated, with an inclusion of second or third choice. Such evidence of omissions in our social welfare and health structures may serve to encourage improvements and therefore should be recorded.

There are repeated examples in which highly competent examinations were nullified by vague, obscure reports replete with esoteric terminology which the court was unable to comprehend or to utilize. As a consequence, the children whom these reports concerned were deprived of vital aid.

When all reports are assembled, the task of evaluation and synthesis completes the main diagnostic process. A high degree of casework skill and understanding is invaluable in assuring that the treatment plan made reflects all that is known about the child and is based upon a practical working knowledge of community resources. The skilled social service worker has an appreciation of the contributions from various fields of specialized knowledge. This, coupled with understanding, helps her to present and interpret the plan to judges and others concerned with the child.

Treatment

Treatment may consist of the following, either singly or in combination: (1) social service counseling and adjustment, including also educational change, such as transfer to a different class, grade, or school; (2) medical care; (3) psychotherapy in a clinic or hospital; (4) placement in a foster home, shelter, or other child-caring institutions; (5) commitment to a correctional or noncorrectional institution or to a state school for the mentally deficient. Selection depends upon the child's needs and capacities as well as upon the availability of various facilities.

Some of the most tragic cases of all represent children or adults of normal intelligence who are inaccessible to treatment in our present state of knowledge. Attention should be focused upon assisting them to become responsive to helpful services. It is hoped that the efficacy of each type of treatment will receive continuous evaluation conducive to steady improvement and progress.

Social casework counseling service may be received within children's courts, guidance clinics, family service agencies, child placement groups, and in the most progressive child-caring and correctional institutions. Any probation or parole system which lacks sufficient casework staff usually fails to accomplish its goals.

Increasingly it is recognized that social workers within juvenile courts have a significant role to play in the realm of treatment, provided they possess the requisite skill together with a practical knowledge of community resources. Often they are able to effect lasting arrangements for the child through individual and group counseling with him, his parents, teachers, and representatives of social and health agencies. On many occasions these adjustment services preclude the necessity for judicial hearings. Voluntary participation of all concerned is an essential ingredient, but the court's authority can be a potent force in stimulating cooperation, especially of parents.

Social service personnel of the court also aid judges before, during and after hearings by gathering and synthesizing pertinent data concerning the child, his family, and the facilities which can be utilized for him. Although certain judges tend to ignore or to minimize treatment plans suggested by social workers, others welcome and apply these in the interest of child offenders. That which appeals to most juvenile court judges is practicality and also simplicity in recommendations.

Close relations between court social service staff, teachers and other educational personnel are as imperative as between social workers and social agencies. Experience demonstrates that many delinquents can be helped materially by transfers to different classes, grades, or schools. When this becomes apparent to the court in specific instances, changes can be effected only by means of cooperative effort with educational authorities. It is here that social workers experienced in school problems are singularly useful in promoting a mutuality of understanding and aims. Definite channelizing systems are as indispensable in this as in other areas of cooperative action for discussion and interchange of information.

Where the court places a child on probation or parole, individual counseling service may form the major treatment plan. In these cases he and his parents usually are referred to a casework agency, and cooperation between the court and agency staffs is of prime importance.

Prompt and complete medical care is vital for many youthful offenders whose physical handicaps in part or in whole have contributed to their misconduct. Ordinarily, service in an outpatient clinic suffices, but at times hospitalization is a necessity. When parents are informed, they generally are quick to provide for medical attention. Where they refuse unreasonably, the court exercises its power of compulsion.

Examples of such refusal are mostly attributable to parental anxieties, emotional imbalance, or religious beliefs. While sympathetic with these conditions, the court is obliged to make the child's welfare paramount by insisting that essential care be furnished him.

The question of psychotherapy is more complicated, first, because it is less understood and, secondly, because facilities are so limited in extent as to become mainly diagnostic centers rather than treatment centers. In fact, even their diagnostic intake has had to be curtailed severely because of staff shortages. To learn that a child or parent needs psychiatric service is significant, but it loses validity if there is no place equipped to render the help.

A fortunate few can afford to pay for prolonged and intensive private psychotherapy. Others, limited to weekly or still more infrequent clinic interviews, become impatient and resistive. Of course it is realized that some patients do not need such intensive or prolonged care as others. But it is found that even several months of concentrated service is usually more efficacious than intermittent interviews over a long period of time.

Additional psychiatric facilities are urgent, so that children and adults who require psychotherapy can obtain it in the community while their problems are still treatable. Psychiatrists agree that the earlier treatment is received the greater chance there is for cure. Failure to receive timely help will mean more serious deviations in the future, with greater suffering and a greater burden upon state hospitals. The consequent loss to the community in human and economic values should not be overlooked.

When a child or his parent is mentally ill either functionally or organically, hospitalization may be required. In this event, remand or commitment to a state institution may be ordered. Such drastic action should be taken only upon a firm foundation of expert examination and opinion. Every effort should be made to assure that youngsters are housed and treated separately from adult mental patients. Concentrated therapy may enable placement with normal children after a short interval.

If a youthful offender is so mentally deficient as to need institutionalization, it can be accomplished by commitment to a state school for the feeble-minded. Although these schools are overcrowded, their officials do the utmost possible for children who are awaiting admission from courts and hospitals. These are among the most hopeless offenders, for there is no way of supplying additional innate intellectual capacity.

Their own protection and that of society demands their placement in special schools where they will receive close supervision and training according to their receptivity. Many sex offenses and crimes of violence are attributable to them and to the group expertly diagnosed as psychopathic personalities.

Effective treatment methods for those termed psychopathic personalities are still in experimental form. Generally speaking, they do not respond well to psychotherapy or social casework counseling. Experience indicates that they are poor risks for either probation or parole, since their rate of recidivism is exceedingly high. For their own welfare and society's, institutionalization is imperative. Every known rehabilitative modus operandi should be attempted, because from this relatively small group stems a substantial number of the most violent and repulsive crimes.

Various types of placement are employed as treatment. A child offender whose home is found to be wholly unsuited to his regeneration has to be removed from it. The question then arises: In what substitute home should he live? A sound answer depends upon two elements: (1) an accurate understanding of his needs and capacities; (2) the availability of placement opportunities.

Relatively few suitable foster homes have been open to delinquent children. By and large they require a period of group living before they are likely to make a satisfactory adjustment in a foster home.

While a brief interval in a shelter has a degree of treatment value for certain offenders, it usually is not a sound placement except as a diagnostic step prior to court hearings in special instances.

Admission to a rehabilitative center such as Hawthorne, Cedar Knolls, or Berkshire Farms often produces constructive results. Their dynamic leadership, trained and interested personnel, wholesome physical surroundings and purposive programs of health, education, guidance, and recreation have made these institutions extraordinarily successful in helping children to new pathways. Significantly enough, each of these has an effective follow-up service which assists graduates in making a transition from institutional life to individual living. Vocational activity and personal counseling are vital phases of this service, which aids materially in reducing the rate of recidivism among these individuals.

Unfortunately, institutions of such high standards are rare and their intake capacity is all too small in comparison with the large number of children who could benefit markedly from their philosophy and methods.

Incredible as it may seem, offenders in New York do not have access to any comparable public centers. This lack is an outgrowth of the well known system of subsidies for private child-caring institutions as a substitute for public care. There has been a fear that public employees would not be so interested and concerned about their charges as religious and charitable groups who have voluntarily pre-empted the field.

As a consequence, there are thousands of private child-caring institutions, each with restrictions upon its admissions, including religion, sex, age, health, grade, scholastic achievement, intelligence level, family conditions, and behavior patterns. Some even adhere to racial qualifications. In New York, and elsewhere too, it is practically impossible to find a placement for a Protestant child offender, especially if he is a Negro. Consequently, either he is returned to an unwholesome home where conditions are conducive to further delinquency, or he is committed to a correctional institution. This is a sad commentary on our present welfare structure.

It cannot be denied that each private group has justification for setting such intake requirements as will enable it to build a unified program for the children it serves and to operate within its limitations of funds and space. Admittedly, it is unsatisfactory to commingle those who are vastly different in age range, intellectual capacity, emotional balance, and habit patterns. But it must also be recognized that each time an eligibility requirement is introduced in addition to the child's need for a substitute home, more children are excluded than included. Hence the necessity for public as well as private programs.

All gradations are found among the private child-caring institutions from the most modern and progressive to antiquated ones still emphasizing custodial care as a major function. Among social workers it is well known that the chief lag in our entire welfare structure is in the field of child care.

Much of this lag results from the persistence of public subsidies for private institutions. Not until government officials accept as a responsibility the provision of modern public care for dependent, neglected, and delinquent children will they discard the outmoded system of subsidies. Rivalries and jealousies among these groups are another harmful element.

Although tax funds are allocated to them, there is little public supervision of their activities aside from the examination of a statistical report and financial accounting. Small wonder it is that archaic operations continue unchecked. Many such institutions are governed by self-perpetuating boards of directors not conversant with modern concepts of child care. Often they do not realize the desirability of trained staff members and high standards of social service.

Since practically all represent religious denominations, there is an understandable reluctance on the part of public officials to inquire into their daily operations. Only when communities become sufficiently aware of the facts will long-delayed changes be made. Expert and impartial evaluation of programs is needed so that treatment through placement can be strengthened and encouraged.

Correctional institutions remain largely places of custodial care rather than of rehabilitation, although some advance has been made in certain of these by the introduction of guidance and other therapeutic services. Studies of the children committed there disclose that the vast majority could be helped to a considerable extent by well planned and well directed programs of health, education, individual guidance, and recreation. When it is considered that all these offenders are released within a few years after their admission, it behooves communities to insist that while there they receive all known rehabilitative care. As it is, many of them graduate to adult criminal courts and penal institutions soon after their release.

Teamwork between children's courts and placement agencies and institutions, also including places of correction, is vital. The resulting interchange of data rebounds to the benefit of juvenile offenders, making their stay of more value. Most of the groups require from the court social summaries of the child, with health and other diagnostic data for use in treatment programs.

The Role of the Schools

In homes and in elementary schools lies the greatest opportunity for the prevention of delinquency. It is incumbent upon educators as well as parents to understand clearly what can be done toward this goal. Practically all the children who later appear in court reveal within their school life indications of maladjustment which can be observed and are susceptible of remedy.

With developments in testing processes, there can be and should be early identification of pupils who are mentally deficient, physically ill, educationally retarded, or suffering from emotional deviations. To accomplish it, there must be less reliance upon group and other cursory examinations and more use of individual tests and measurements administered by qualified examiners together with skilled individual counseling.

Since feeble-mindedness can be ascertained in the primary grades by means of psychometric study, there is little excuse for retaining imbecilic students year after year until their often precocious physical development and lack of control find expression in misconduct that is harmful to schoolmates and themselves. The sooner their exact mental status is determined and provision is made for their transfer to other schools equipped to deal with them, the better off they and the other pupils will be. The cost of additional psychologists to identify these children will be offset many times over by savings in human and property damage.

Similarly, full medical study of every pupil will disclose those with correctable physical defects. Except in rare instances, parental cooperation can be obtained in securing essential medical service either privately, in clinics, or hospitals. If it is not forthcoming, compulsive methods must be resorted to for the child's sake. Perfunctory notations of the same physical problem on the student's health record card are not enough. In other words, the discovery of medical defect should be followed through by school authorities to see that remedial attention is obtained.

With the advances made in medical science there is no excuse for uncorrected childhood conditions of impaired vision or hearing, dental caries, diseased respiratory systems, and other ailments.

Educational retardation among elementary pupils and its causes are readily ascertainable by competent psychologists. The longer it persists, the more extensive it grows, with the result that school becomes utterly distasteful. School frustrations intensify and multiply emotional conflicts that have developed because of unstable home conditions. Children who are misgraded and thus unable to keep up with their classmates and those who have little aptitude or interest in academic subjects flee from school. While idle and unsupervised, they become involved in delinquent acts.

Automatic grade promotions regardless of class achievement tend to promote scholastic disabilities. Many examples are found in which pupils with reading and arithmetic scores of 3A have been promoted automatically each semester until they reached junior high school, where they could not begin to cope successfully with their studies. In despair they truanted and misbehaved in other ways. Naturally, it is not recommended that students be failed repeatedly and retained in classes with much younger ones; that, too, is an unsound solution, for it also creates problems—bullying, humiliations, and attempts to escape school attendance.

Surely there must be a course in between these two extremes with focus upon the causal elements occasioning school failures and upon methods of prevention and cure. Each of these extremes is an injustice to the child and a source of future trouble for him, the school, and in many instances for the community as well.

Deviations in the emotional sphere can also be determined during the elementary years. Even incipient or actual mental illness among children is usually discernible before they reach high school. Teachers who possess a knowledge and understanding of fundamental mental hygiene concepts can help in the identification process. Smaller classes with more individual attention for students will also aid. Analysis of Rorschach patterns by qualified psychologists as an essential part of all psychometric studies will cast light upon serious emotional disturbances.

Social workers assigned to elementary schools can play an important role by offering individual counseling service to parents and pupils and by conferences and discussions with teachers, singly and in groups.

Caseworkers are trained to diagnose cases of incipient delinquency and maladjustment. They can help parents to accept a child's difficulty and to plan for treatment before it reaches an acute stage. Most parents are willing and able to improve their handling of their children if competent and timely assistance is given them. Often they do not realize the destructive effect of certain attitudes and patterns within the home until it is explained and interpreted.

Where more complete study or treatment is desirable, school social workers can make cooperative arrangements with clinics, guidance units, family service agencies, and placement groups.

It has rightly been said that parent education should begin in early childhood, not in adulthood, since that which makes for emotional maturity is the best possible training for parenthood. Besides aiding pupils to mental health, elementary schools could well become centers of parent education. Educational personnel have a natural entree to parents within the neighborhood and thus have an opportunity to reach more families than any social agency, public or private.

A tactful, understanding approach is essential; both content and method should be geared to the parents themselves, their degree of education, capacity, and receptivity. It is encouraging to note the large percentage who welcome occasions for the discussion of common problems, doubts, and perplexities concerning their children. Group meetings on a highly practical level supplemented by individual counseling would be salutary and would constitute a valuable contribution to sound community relations.

If parent-teacher organizations could be transformed into genuine parent education groups under dynamic leadership, a major step forward would be made in the prevention of juvenile delinquency. Stress upon voluntary sharing in the programs is suggested, with no compulsion or pressure. The wealth of authentic case material at hand could be translated readily into nontechnical terms. With lively presentation, these group discussions could prove as absorbing as most of the daytime radio features which attract large audiences.

It is a hopeful sign when schools reach out to the public instead of holding aloof. Our educational systems are integral parts of community life, and wholesome growth is possible only if there is a recognition of this principle, especially in a democracy. Schools can teach democracy best by practicing it and sharing in the development of healthful parenthood.

Variation in curricula within elementary and junior high schools is sadly lacking. Traditionally, subject matter has been restricted to academic subjects with a scattering of classes in domestic arts and shop which few take very seriously. Yet, as has been pointed out previously, a substantial proportion of children who develop patterns of misconduct do so partly as a result of distaste for school engendered by a disinterest in and little capacity for academic studies.

Pupils who are vocationally inclined are expected to enter vocational schools, but these are practically all high schools with strict requirements for admission, including graduation from an elementary school or its equivalent, average intelligence, special aptitude, and interest. Vocational high schools are a valuable part of our educational framework, meeting the needs of thousands of children, but such schools are not the solution for the vast numbers of those who can never qualify for entrance nor master a skilled trade. It should be borne in mind that nonacademic interests are not equivalent to a high degree of manual dexterity, although the two sometimes go together.

Many pupils could be taught the semiskilled and simple trades within elementary and junior high schools with lasting benefit to themselves, their families, and society. Otherwise, when they reach 16 they drop out of school, lacking even rudimentary skills, and swell the ranks of the unemployed. In the age group from 16 to 21 there is found the highest ratio of penal offenses, especially crimes of violence.

Insufficient vocational training in these schools represents a very serious social lag which educators have a duty to remedy without further delay. In doing so they will be making a vital contribution toward a stable society.

More remedial instruction, coupled with skilled individual counseling and guidance services, would also assist materially in the sphere of prevention and treatment. These efforts would be strengthened by flexibility in arranging transfers to different grades, classes, and schools when recommended by experts. Teachers, principals, and other personnel can facilitate or hinder a course of treatment in court, clinic, or social agency by their attitudes and actions. While most are eager to be helpful, others become emotionally involved, at times to the point of a personal feud with the pupil.

Two cases may serve as illustrations. One concerns Albert, who while under clinic care returned to school, resolved to behave himself. When the aid of his principal was sought, the response was, "Help that boy? I'll help him to jail!" When Stephen, also receiving psychotherapy, went back to school his principal, incensed at previous truancies, refused to sign a class permit. After Stephen was kept waiting in the principal's office for three days he left school and refused to return.

School expulsions also merit comment. Where a student's misbehavior reaches such proportions as to warrant his exclusion, undoubtedly there were prior manifestations of maladjustment which should have received competent study and treatment. Perhaps then there would not have been a need for such drastic action in a considerable number of instances. When a pupil is barred, little is accomplished if the school's concern ends with his ejection.

Certain students welcome expulsion as freedom from the exactions of school and proceed to roam the streets or frequent poolrooms, etc. Unless prompt action follows they soon become implicated in unlawful acts. Their parents tend to become confused and defensive, blaming the school and shielding the child.

Expulsion cases are sometimes referred to children's court by pressure from district superintendents who realize that these children need help, not punishment. Scrutiny reveals that many are suffering from extreme mental deficiency or grave emotional disturbance at times verging on mental illness or brain disorder. For each, skilled diagnosis and treatment are indispensable.

Attendance bureaus are in a strategic position to assist in the field of prevention and treatment, provided they are capably staffed. They encounter incipient and actual delinquents at the onset of their careers when help is still timely. Truant officers also have opportunity to discover neglected children whose parents have permitted them or even encouraged them to remain at home or to accept unlawful work.

While the battle over function rages, fundamentally the attendance job is social casework, as shown in the preceding cases and others as well. Its police aspects are only auxiliary. Employment of qualified social service personnel is essential to carry out attendance duties such as social study of the truant and his family, counseling and lasting adjustments, together with purposive referrals to social and health agencies and courts.

New York City lags behind other communities in the quality of its attendance work, largely because of a failure to assign caseworkers as truant officers. Emphasis upon police functions and punitive measures joined with amateur social service result in constant repetitions of the same cases. Incomplete and inadequate records are also grave handicaps, since continuity and comprehensiveness of social records are a prerequisite to effective work with individuals and families.

Moreover, the New York City Bureau of Attendance usually does not utilize social service exchange data at the start of difficult cases. Instead, it waits until court action is contemplated. It does so then only under pressure from the court. By this delay the Bureau deprives itself of available information which is exceedingly valuable in planning for children. That is one reason why its administrative hearings are so often ineffectual.

A multiplicity of these hearings is also characteristic of the Bureau's program. Long delays ensue, causing pupils to become more set in their habits of truancy. Frequently the hearings are nothing more than repetitious recitals of names, addresses, absence dates, and the child's prolonged truancy. There is no justification for a perpetuation of such duplication. No legislation is necessary to effect a change; administrative action by the Board of Education would suffice.

It is only fair to mention that on occasion some staff members of this Bureau achieve excellent adjustments and make productive referrals to social and health agencies. But these are the exception rather than the rule and are brought about despite, not because of, existing leadership.

Probationary and parental schools offer fruitful topics for discussion. To the former, pupils who are considered serious disciplinary problems and habitual truants may be transferred from neighborhood schools while they continue to reside at home. Although figures are submitted indicating improved attendance records, these are not always a true index, since some of the pupils are escorted almost daily by truant officers. A few vocational subjects are taught, and more individual attention is received along with remedial instruction and a degree of guidance. There is also a high degree of cooperation with clinics and courts where many of the students are under treatment.

The high incidence of recidivism among probationary school pupils implies that the value of these schools is questionable. It would seem far more sound to equip neighborhood schools with flexible curricula, experienced caseworkers, and other counseling personnel and to retain those children who are not in need of institutionalization.

Those who are shown by careful study to be for the most part normal but require a period of rehabilitation away from home might well be placed in a parental school that is geared to their needs. The term "youth center" would be descriptive of its functions. It is true that certain parental schools fell into disrepute because of staff inadequacies. But this should not prejudice a community against the concept of parental schools.

Most modern educational systems contain qualified teachers, group workers, caseworkers, psychologists, psychiatrists, physicians, and nurses. From these could be selected the requisite personnel to establish and operate treatment centers where these children could receive intensive care. The duration of their stay would be an individual matter depending upon the circumstances of each case. Some children might be helped sufficiently in a week, while others might productively remain a semester.

It would appear wise to review each periodically and thoroughly. If more than a semester's residence is suggested for a child, perhaps another type of placement might be advisable.

Who should decide which pupils are to be placed in such a youth center? Juvenile courts might well be given this task rather than individuals within the educational system. The court is in an intermediary position between the family and the school. It can resist pressures from either side and more readily bear the onus of responsibility and complaint because it would be recognized as an impartial body.

Children's Courts

For the most part, the legal foundation upon which these judicial bodies rest is broad and liberal. There is both an expressed and implied intent that the court shall exist to protect and to benefit children who come within its scope. Detailed provision is made for jurisdiction and powers, structure, practice and procedure, records, staff, and other matters. Since these courts are created by legislative enactment, the rule of strict statutory construction applies, especially as to jurisdiction and powers. But as to daily activities, there is opportunity for more liberal interpretation than is sometimes exercised by timorous personnel.

Jurisdiction is limited mainly to children under 16 who are alleged to be either dependent, neglected, or delinquent. Although each of these terms is specifically defined, human situations are not so rigidly classifiable. Hence, there remain those who do not fall into the three groupings yet who need the court's aid. Unfortunately, it is powerless to assist them. A few judges, in their anxiety to be of service, expand the definitions, but realize that should their decisions be challenged by writ or appeal they would be overruled and perhaps censored by higher tribunals.

Generally speaking, a dependent child is one who is without financial support, whereas a neglected child is one without proper guardianship or lacking in physical care, which is considered to include also medical attention. Recently there has been a slight tendency to extend the concept of neglect to include emotional deprivation. Although this is more realistic in many instances, can it validly be said that a parent is neglectful for not accepting psychotherapy when, like many other people, he does not understand its value or significance?

If a child's misconduct is not serious, a neglect petition may be taken instead of a delinquency one. Two reasons account for the practice. One is to avoid stigmatizing him; the other is that few constructive placements are available for delinquents. However, if there is no evidence of neglect but he needs the court's help to obtain special care, he may be labeled a delinquent.

While it is recognized that limitations have to be placed upon the jurisdiction and powers of courts, nevertheless, it would be worth while to include a fourth category. Where judicial action is required for a child's welfare, the court should be permitted to proceed. Appeals and writs would be remedies against arbitrary decisions. To effect a change legislation would be necessary.

Despite the fact that children's courts aid many thousands of dependent and neglected youngsters, the picture as to delinquents is not so encouraging. In fairness it should be remembered that the latter cases usually are more complex, although often the line of demarcation between neglect and delinquency is exceedingly tenuous. The large number of children reappearing in court exemplify certain weaknesses.

The first and most pointed is the lack of judges trained and experienced in the problems of childhood. Almost invariably they are sincere and eager to do their utmost, but good intentions and zeal are not enough to cope successfully with the difficult cases presented. The best of probation work can be nullified by inept judicial opinions. It is destructive for children and families and disheartening for the staff when careful study and practical treatment plans are negated. Other staff members must then try to rectify matters, for almost always in such cases nothing has been solved. It is not suggested that the judge should accept recommendations and opinions uncritically. But he should be adequately equipped to evaluate these accurately, inasmuch as he has the responsibility for decisions.

No substantial progress will be made in these courts until judicial appointments cease to be political. Social welfare organizations and other community groups have a duty to take more interest and to be more actively concerned in the selection of juvenile court judges. Instead of waiting passively for them to be chosen and then lamenting the choice, these bodies should seek out qualified individuals and work cooperatively towards their appointment. Not until its judges possess specialized training and experience amounting to expertness in the problems of children will a juvenile court take its place in the community as a social agency geared to meet childhood's needs.

A stronger probation staff is another prime requisite. While considerable improvement has been achieved in the past decade, much remains to be done. Salaries are so low that many of the younger, better qualified officers are transferring to other positions. Qualifications should be raised along with salaries. Professional training is as indispensable here as in a family service agency or child-caring institution. An alert in-service training program under dynamic leadership would prove valuable. Each probation unit should be sufficiently manned so that there can be thorough study of all intake together with prompt service after initial hearings. The better equipped the probation units are, the greater the number of satisfactory adjustments that are possible, with or without judicial proceedings.

Juvenile courts should adopt a more understanding role in counseling with parents, particularly on the question of involuntary commitments. Court personnel should be alert and responsive to the opportunities for service in this area.

More qualitative research and evaluation are needed to test the efficacy of both study and treatment methods. Statistical reports are useful but do not give a true picture of strengths and weaknesses. The value of qualitative research for administrative purposes and for the extension of social knowledge should receive more emphasis.

A vigorous public relations policy is imperative in explaining the problems and the work of the court. It should be remembered that public support is a prerequisite to obtaining the additional clinical and placement facilities which are so sorely needed. Waiting until the court is under attack before furnishing information and interpretation is negativistic and harmful.

Although the School Part of the New York City Children's Court has been valuable as an experiment in the realm of prevention and treatment, the writer is convinced that its program should be merged with that of other divisions, as truancy and school misconduct are not fundamentally separable from other symptoms of maladjustment such as stealing, sex offenses, etc. In the interests of children structural and functional integration is imperative.

In New York City the Children's Court is further handicapped by lack of a central index and by a system of rotating judicial assignments. As it is, a child may be known to one branch while his family may be known to another, without an interchange of data or an integrated plan. Likewise, the same child may be dealt with separately in two different sections. Since there is no single registry of all cases, duplications and overlappings are discovered only by accident. That this is shortsighted and costly both in human and economic terms needs no elaboration. It is hoped that an administrative change will be made without further delay.

Rotation of judges results in more than one presiding over the same case because more than one hearing is usually scheduled. Since only the barest notations are inscribed on petitions, it follows that succeeding judges generally are unaware of what has transpired and must approach the problem anew. Repetitious testimony is given and further delays occur, sometimes with devastating effects upon those whom the court is trying to assist. Moreover, these shifts often make it impossible for judges to test the value of their own methods and decisions, as mistakes are left for other judges to correct, if possible, on the adjourned dates. Continuity of approach is peculiarly important in the handling of children's cases.

Social Agencies

As the significant role of social agencies has been implicit throughout this volume, only brief comment is made here. These agencies and their workers have been instrumental in the passage of welfare legislation, including that creating juvenile courts. Yet, they are inclined to overlook the fact that no law, however well formulated and basically sound, is self-executing, but depends upon the caliber of the personnel administering it. Therefore, social agencies should concern themselves more with the court's daily functioning. The necessity of modifications, both legislative and in administrative practices, is revealed in day by day operations.

More flexible intake policies would be desirable, especially among the placement groups. It is sometimes forgotten that flexibility in intake is fully as productive as flexibility in the under-care case load. If only they would pool their facilities in favor of the total number of youngsters needing substitute homes, for the present placement situation is tragic in its implications!

Social workers should have a first-hand knowledge of shelters, rehabilitative centers, places of correction, state schools for the mentally deficient, and hospitals for the mentally ill. By visiting such institutions they will be better prepared to counsel with parents and children.

It is recommended that social agencies make more use of cooperative systems and methods for channelizing the interchange of data and suggestions. Changes which are based upon sifted field experience are likely to prove workable. Continuous evaluation of program and activities is also beneficial. In this connection, planned administrative research helps to bring about purposive change. When evaluation and research are accompanied by timely and comprehensive interpretation, there is a resulting gain in public support.

Social agencies and their staff members have an obligation to furnish leadership in meeting the challenge to community organization which demands a maximum use of existing facilities, together with additional ones so that many thousands of child offenders may be helped to lead productive lives.

Patterson Smith Reprint Series in Criminology, Law Enforcement, and Social Problems

1. Lewis: *The Development of American Prisons and Prison Customs, 1776-1845*
2. Carpenter: *Reformatory Prison Discipline*
3. Brace: *The Dangerous Classes of New York*
4. Dix: *Remarks on Prisons and Prison Discipline in the United States*
5. Bruce et al: *The Workings of the Indeterminate-Sentence Law and the Parole System in Illinois*
6. Wickersham Commission: *Complete Reports, Including the Mooney-Billings Report.* 14 Vols.
7. Livingston: *Complete Works on Criminal Jurisprudence.* 2 Vols.
8. Cleveland Foundation: *Criminal Justice in Cleveland*
9. Illinois Association for Criminal Justice: *The Illinois Crime Survey*
10. Missouri Association for Criminal Justice: *The Missouri Crime Survey*
11. Aschaffenburg: *Crime and Its Repression*
12. Garofalo: *Criminology*
13. Gross: *Criminal Psychology*
14. Lombroso: *Crime, Its Causes and Remedies*
15. Saleilles: *The Individualization of Punishment*
16. Tarde: *Penal Philosophy*
17. McKelvey: *American Prisons*
18. Sanders: *Negro Child Welfare in North Carolina*
19. Pike: *A History of Crime in England.* 2 Vols.
20. Herring: *Welfare Work in Mill Villages*
21. Barnes: *The Evolution of Penology in Pennsylvania*
22. Puckett: *Folk Beliefs of the Southern Negro*
23. Fernald et al: *A Study of Women Delinquents in New York State*
24. Wines: *The State of the Prisons and of Child-Saving Institutions*
25. Raper: *The Tragedy of Lynching*
26. Thomas: *The Unadjusted Girl*
27. Jorns: *The Quakers as Pioneers in Social Work*
28. Owings: *Women Police*
29. Woolston: *Prostitution in the United States*
30. Flexner: *Prostitution in Europe*
31. Kelso: *The History of Public Poor Relief in Massachusetts: 1820-1920*
32. Spivak: *Georgia Nigger*
33. Earle: *Curious Punishments of Bygone Days*
34. Bonger: *Race and Crime*
35. Fishman: *Crucibles of Crime*
36. Brearley: *Homicide in the United States*
37. Graper: *American Police Administration*
38. Hichborn: *"The System"*
39. Steiner & Brown: *The North Carolina Chain Gang*
40. Cherrington: *The Evolution of Prohibition in the United States of America*
41. Colquhoun: *A Treatise on the Commerce and Police of the River Thames*
42. Colquhoun: *A Treatise on the Police of the Metropolis*
43. Abrahamsen: *Crime and the Human Mind*
44. Schneider: *The History of Public Welfare in New York State: 1609-1866*
45. Schneider & Deutsch: *The History of Public Welfare in New York State: 1867-1940*
46. Crapsey: *The Nether Side of New York*
47. Young: *Social Treatment in Probation and Delinquency*
48. Quinn: *Gambling and Gambling Devices*
49. McCord & McCord: *Origins of Crime*
50. Worthington & Topping: *Specialized Courts Dealing with Sex Delinquency*

PATTERSON SMITH REPRINT SERIES IN CRIMINOLOGY, LAW ENFORCEMENT, AND SOCIAL PROBLEMS

51. Asbury: *Sucker's Progress*
52. Kneeland: *Commercialized Prostitution in New York City*
53. Fosdick: *American Police Systems*
54. Fosdick: *European Police Systems*
55. Shay: *Judge Lynch: His First Hundred Years*
56. Barnes: *The Repression of Crime*
57. Cable: *The Silent South*
58. Kammerer: *The Unmarried Mother*
59. Doshay: *The Boy Sex Offender and His Later Career*
60. Spaulding: *An Experimental Study of Psychopathic Delinquent Women*
61. Brockway: *Fifty Years of Prison Service*
62. Lawes: *Man's Judgment of Death*
63. Healy & Healy: *Pathological Lying, Accusation, and Swindling*
64. Smith: *The State Police*
65. Adams: *Interracial Marriage in Hawaii*
66. Halpern: *A Decade of Probation*
67. Tappan: *Delinquent Girls in Court*
68. Alexander & Healy: *Roots of Crime*
69. Healy & Bronner: *Delinquents and Criminals*
70. Cutler: *Lynch-Law*
71. Gillin: *Taming the Criminal*
72. Osborne: *Within Prison Walls*
73. Ashton: *The History of Gambling in England*
74. Whitlock: *On the Enforcement of Law in Cities*
75. Goldberg: *Child Offenders*
76. Cressey: *The Taxi-Dance Hall*
77. Riis: *The Battle with the Slum*
78. Larson *et al: Lying and Its Detection*
79. Comstock: *Frauds Exposed*
80. Carpenter: *Our Convicts.* 2 Vols. in 1
81. Horn: *Invisible Empire: The Story of the Ku Klux Klan, 1866-1871*
82. Faris *et al: Intelligent Philanthropy*
83. Robinson: *History and Organization of Criminal Statistics in the United States*
84. Reckless: *Vice in Chicago*
85. Healy: *The Individual Delinquent*
86. Bogen: *Jewish Philanthropy*
87. Clinard: *The Black Market: A Study of White Collar Crime*
88. Healy: *Mental Conflicts and Misconduct*
89. Citizens' Police Committee: *Chicago Police Problems*
90. Clay: *The Prison Chaplain*
91. Peirce: *A Half Century with Juvenile Delinquents*
92. Richmond: *Friendly Visiting Among the Poor*
93. Brasol: *Elements of Crime*
94. Strong: *Public Welfare Administration in Canada*
95. Beard: *Juvenile Probation*
96. Steinmetz: *The Gaming Table.* 2 Vols.
97. Crawford: *Report on the Penitentiaries of the United States*
98. Kuhlman: *A Guide to Material on Crime and Criminal Justice*
99. Culver: *Bibliography of Crime and Criminal Justice: 1927-1931*
100. Culver: *Bibliography of Crime and Criminal Justice: 1932-1937*